"*The Mind-Body Stress Reset* provides clear theoretical and practical guidance to help people restore their vital capacity for resilience in the aftermath of trauma and toxic stress. It does this through simple, well-conceived tools employing body awareness. This book is equally valuable for new therapists, accomplished ones, and to all of those seeking inner balance and wholeness."

—**Peter A. Levine, PhD**, founder of Somatic Experiencing®, and author of *Waking the Tiger* and *In an Unspoken Voice*

"Like a good friend who knows the territory through hard-won personal experience, Rebekkah LaDyne shows that you have everything you need for well-being right inside of you. Written in an engaging, accessible style, *The Mind-Body Stress Reset* offers simple yet profound science-based tools that train you to self-regulate your stress and connect with your optimal self. You don't have to go down the rabbit hole of your mind. You can learn how to connect with the wisdom of the body that helps you be grounded and not miss the blessing of being alive. A truly excellent contribution."

—**James Baraz, MA,** cofounding teacher at Spirit Rock Meditation Center, and coauthor of *Awakening Joy*

"*The Mind-Body Stress Reset* does just what the title claims. Drawing deeply from the traditions of somatics, yoga, mindfulness, and contemporary research, Rebekkah LaDyne presents a pragmatic and user-friendly approach to addressing stress in a way that is accessible, useful, and effective!"

—**Mariana Caplan, PhD, MFT**, author of *Yoga and Psyche* and *Eyes Wide Open*

"I highly recommend Rebekkah LaDyne's book for anyone who has ever experienced anxiety, worry, and tension. Here is a practical guide for enhancing well-being by building resilience. Her approach is well supported by research on somatic therapies and mind-body medicine. LaDyne shows readers effective skills to 'reset' their mind-body baseline. She challenges us to try the skill exercises and achieve a mind-body reset in our lives."

> —**Donald Moss, PhD**, dean of the college of integrative medicine and health sciences at Saybrook University, coauthor of *Pathways to Illness* and *Pathways to Health*, and author of *Integrative Pathways*

"A highly readable manual for life! Offering simple yet effective exercises and surveys to identify and survive modern-day stresses. Creatively written with an excellent mixture of science, research, and self-disclosure, all of which give credibility and depth to Rebekkah LaDyne's knowledge. I highly recommend."

> —**Ariel Giarretto, LMFT, SEP**, Somatic Experiencing® Trauma Institute senior faculty, and internationally recognized somatic psychotherapist

"In an accessible and easy-to-follow way, Rebekkah LaDyne has given the lay reader a clear way to understand stress responses and how to manage them with simple, straightforward strategies. With lightly humorous writing, LaDyne provides a researched overview that should capture readers' creative imaginations to reduce their stress reactions with helpful checklists and exercises that can be done anywhere. The science that supports her writing and ideas is described simply, and will make all readers comfortable in trying the suggestions she offers."

> —**Dave Berger, MFT, PT, SEP**, Somatic Experiencing® Trauma Institute senior faculty, and internationally recognized somatic psychotherapist

"Rebekkah LaDyne combines three powerful and evocative tools: the mental, emotional, and somatic aspects of the human body as long-lasting, natural defenses against stress in a sometimes-chaotic world. By hacking the mind-body connection in concert, her well-supported methods recognize that the body also needs a voice in maintaining balance. It is with joy and respect that I recommend her book to those of us that need help in remembering that balance."

—**Elena Gillespie, PhD**, adjunct faculty of mind-body medicine at Saybrook University, and author of *The Anatomy of Death*

"Rebekkah LaDyne has written a wise, practical, and insightful guide to working with adversity and stress. Weaving relevant theory with evidence-based practice, LaDyne offers a powerful road map for safe and transformative body-based practice. It is clearly written, full of heart, and an outstanding contribution to the field."

—**David Treleaven, PhD**, author of *Trauma-Sensitive Mindfulness*

"Somatic intelligence is often a neglected or rather forgotten territory. Rebekkah LaDyne shows us with her remarkable book how much potential for healing opens up once we invite this intelligence into our consciousness, and give it space to balance out the wounds of trauma and neglect. The book is a wonderful blend of scientifically based theory and playful exercises. I wish the whole world would read it—I see it as a guide into health, happiness, and joyful living."

—**Urs Honauer, PhD, SEP**, Somatic Experiencing® Trauma Institute senior faculty, and director of the Center for Inner Ecology in Zurich, Switzerland

The

Mind-Body
Stress
Reset

Somatic Practices to Reduce Overwhelm
and Increase Well-Being

REBEKKAH LaDYNE, MS, SEP

New Harbinger Publications, Inc.

Publisher's Note

This publication is designed to provide accurate and authoritative information in regard to the subject matter covered. It is sold with the understanding that the publisher is not engaged in rendering psychological, financial, legal, or other professional services. If expert assistance or counseling is needed, the services of a competent professional should be sought.

All names of clients in this book have been changed to protect anonymity and many of the persons depicted are composites.

NEW HARBINGER PUBLICATIONS is a registered trademark of New Harbinger Publications, Inc.

Distributed in Canada by Raincoast Books

Copyright © 2020 by Rebekkah LaDyne
        New Harbinger Publications, Inc.
        5674 Shattuck Avenue
        Oakland, CA 94609
        www.newharbinger.com

Cover design by Amy Daniel

Illustrations by Hayden Foell

Acquired by Elizabeth Hollis Hansen

Edited by Kristi Hein

All Rights Reserved

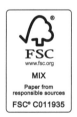

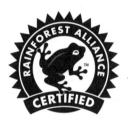

Library of Congress Cataloging-in-Publication Data on file

Printed in the United States of America

24   23   22

10   9   8   7   6   5   4   3   2

Contents

Foreword

Stress is universal. At some point in our lives, nearly every one of us will experience some form of stress. Fortunately, most of us will recover from our stress experiences. However, for some of us stress becomes a more constant companion—we are *not* recovering from our stress experiences. Alarmingly, the percentage of those who fit in that second category is growing. As Rebekkah notes in her introduction to this book, we can accurately say that stress is an epidemic which is getting worse, not better.

Extreme or chronic stress can have a devastating impact on our ability to be in the world in the way we would like. It can extinguish our creativity, our interest in connection, and our ability to manage our own body responses. It can also contribute to a multitude of physical and emotional symptoms.

Stress is not just in our minds. Stress is deeply somatic—that is, it influences us physiologically in ways that can feel beyond our conscious control. Stress creates ingrained somatic "habits" that become very difficult to change—a kind of automatic response system which influences how we respond to our environment, even how we experience our sense of self. This stress response system can become our default system, often creating responses even before we are consciously aware of what's happening. Our mind is following along behind our somatic responses, not leading them.

One of the frustrating things about this type of stress system is that we often have quite a lot of cognitive awareness and understanding of it and of the things that trigger it—and yet, we can't *think* our way out of it. We may even know what needs to change, but are at sea about how to accomplish that change. In my experience of working with many thousands of people who suffer from varying degrees of stress, true change requires a method that includes the body—our somatic self—rather than trying to override or suppress its responses.

The Mind-Body Stress Reset provides tools for doing exactly that. It provides a clear road map for embodying change in our stress responses. Through the simple and straightforward methods presented in this book, we can learn the somatic tools to help us make the transition from chronic stress to embodied resilience. The tools presented here are available to us 24 hours a day. We don't need to go somewhere special to practice them, we can work at our own pace, and we can make real changes in our somatic responses by practicing the methods presented here.

This is one of those rare books that is much, much better than it needed to be. It could have been a simple description of a very effective stress relief protocol: the Mind-Body Stress Reset tools. It would have been a very useful book, and well worth writing. But Rebekkah has gone so much farther than that. She is providing accessible information about the science behind our stress responses and how we can alter those responses to build greater stress resilience. She has provided illustrative stories about how the symptoms of extreme and chronic stress can manifest, and how successes in changing those symptoms can come about. She has also provided very helpful information about the transition from stress to resilience, which provides an excellent guide to how the journey toward resilience may look and feel. Included in this material is information about how we can assess when we may need professional help in addressing our stress symptoms, and when we are likely to be able to make progress on our own.

And that just gets us started on the well-being journey. After a thorough grounding in the foundational material, Rebekkah then provides a well-structured and practical tool kit for step-by-step movement toward change. The methods are clearly articulated, well-researched and based on her direct experience in using them not only for herself, but also for her clients.

As an additional bonus, Rebekkah has provided us with somatic skill-building practices, built directly into the book. At regular intervals, she invites us to take a moment and notice—right now—how we can be in better somatic relationship to ourselves, notice our responses, and apply our somatic awareness to support change in our stress systems.

Over and over again, this book produces that delightful experience of thinking, *Ah, there's a jewel—something I didn't expect, but that is just perfect.* It's a pleasure to read a book that is so wonderfully crafted, which can be an aid not only to those struggling with stress themselves, but also for professionals who are supporting their clients in this change process.

For those who have been suffering from the side effects of extreme or chronic stress, this is a very hope-filled book. You will hear success stories about those who have made substantial recovery from their stress symptoms, and you will be given effective methods to begin that same journey yourself. For those professionals who work with clients or patients whose stress symptoms can benefit from daily somatic practices for building stress resilience, this book is an invaluable source for those practices.

I wish you all well in your healing journeys.

—Kathy L. Kain, PhD

CHAPTER 1

From Extreme Stress to Relief

This is a book about the effects of stress on our minds *and bodies,* and what we can do to help ourselves recover from these effects. Many of us desperately need a new approach to stress reduction, as our previous attempts haven't lifted enough of the strain. This book offers a new approach—a somatic approach. So before we even begin with the thinking part, let's start with the body. Read through these instructions and then try the exercise. w

Beginning with Your Body

I invite you to make yourself as comfortable as possible, right here, wherever you are. Whether you are sitting, standing, or lying down, is there a way you can let yourself settle in *just a bit* more? No pressure, no expectation, only an invitation.

What happens if you pay attention to wherever your body is making contact with the surface you're touching? Where are you being supported or held up? Perhaps by a couch, a bed, the floor? Can you allow that surface to hold you up *just a bit* more, so that you don't have to do quite as much work? Can you receive the simple support that is available there, letting your feet, hips, or back sink into that support? Notice if there are any areas in your body that are holding tension, that do not really need to be tense. Can you invite any of those areas to soften *a bit?* And can your more-relaxed areas give any internal support to your less-relaxed areas?

Last, what if you let your breath be invited to fill your lungs. No need to make it happen, just making room for your breath to breathe itself. Can you let yourself settle with your relaxed breathing here for just a moment?

And now sense this moment just as it is, just as you are. I'm so glad you've arrived here with this book in your hand. Let's begin to explore stress resilience.

STRESS TOUCHES EVERYONE'S LIFE

Whether you've gone through one big stress event or lived through daily stresses that have accumulated over years, you could have stress residue inside you. This residue may be affecting your daily functioning. Stress might be dictating how you feel, think, and act, at work, at home, with family, and with friends.

It turns out that stress is a big issue that many of us suffer from. At the time of this writing, 78 percent of adults say they suffer from stress and 24 percent of adults report suffering from *extreme* stress. Recent surveys convey that more than forty million adults suffer from anxiety, which is stress in a different outfit. Stress and anxiety are both forms of stress reactivity. What's more, we're getting more stressed—data show that each subsequent generation reports suffering from *greater* stress levels than the previous generation. From "matures" to boomers, Gen Xers to millennials, each generation is more afflicted with overwhelm, worry, and fear than the one before.

With regard to stress, instead of evolving, we seem to be devolving—it's as if stress is an epidemic, or more likely a pandemic. The symptoms of this epi/pandemic come in all shapes and sizes. Feeling stranded in states of overwhelm, stress, and anxiety is keeping us up at night; impeding our digestion and elimination; inducing headaches and joint pains; eroding our relationships; distracting us at work; and even wreaking havoc on our immune systems, making us ill. This stress is also making us anxious: anxious at work, anxious when not at work, anxious at home, anxious when away from home, anxious about being with people, anxious about being alone, anxious, anxious, anxious. Unfortunately, the frequency with which we *experience* and *enact* stress is creating what we could call deep stress imprints. These imprints are like maps our body-mind system follows in the face of stress, and these maps can repeatedly lead us toward deep insecurities and fears about countless aspects of our lives.

Explore This: Does stress show up in your life?

Assign a number from 1 to 10 to each life circumstance,
1 being very little stress, 10 being extreme stress.

Where and when do you feel stressed?			
_____	At work?	_____	At home?
_____	When socializing?	_____	When alone?
_____	In your romantic relationship(s)?	_____	When out of a romantic relationship?
_____	With friends?	_____	With family?
_____	When traveling afar?	_____	When in your home city or town?
_____	When the pace of life is fast and full?	_____	When life is going slow and sparse?
_____	Regarding your health (physical, mental, emotional)?	_____	Regarding self-care (exercise, diet, personal time...)?
_____	With peers?	_____	With superiors?
_____	Regarding money?	_____	Regarding physical safety?
_____	Concerning the past?	_____	Concerning the future?
_____	Other _____	_____	Other _____

IS IT ALL ME, OR DID I INHERIT
SOME OF THIS?

There *is* an evolutionary basis for all of this stress. I fondly say that we are the descendants of the most hypervigilant, anxious, and stressed humans there ever were. Back in prehistoric times, the humans who were chilling out watching a beautiful sunset instead of committedly (or neurotically) scanning for danger, were not *eating* dinner later; they *were* dinner.

Our ancient ancestors—the ones who survived, anyway—had to be incredibly aware of possible threats, always on the lookout for what was coming next, and always rehearsing how to survive the bad stuff that was *surely* just ahead (wink, wink; *of course* the hypervigilant would assume that ruin was imminent). They also must have spent a lot of time rehashing the bad stuff that had just happened so as to avoid it next time. This genetic inheritance makes for an extremely adept survival brain, which is very good at stress reactivity. After all, we've been rehearsing and rehashing our stress reactions for thousands upon thousands of years.

Don't get me wrong. I'm incredibly grateful that our ancient ancestors were so hypervigilant. But this has also left us with a heavy load, an intense predisposition for stress reactivity and its friends, overwhelm and anxiety. Taking this predisposition back to the metaphor of stress pathways in the body-mind might look something like this: with years of evolution and our current day-to-day stresses, our stress-reactivity pathways are like well-engineered autobahns whose onramps have flashing signs reading "Enter Here."

For the regularly stressed, these autobahns of stress are our familiar routes; they are so familiar that they're easy to return to again and again. These stress routes are fast and efficient, even a little thrilling, but the tolls from this travel are very, very high. Meanwhile, our routes to recover from stress—I'll call them our *resilience pathways*—are what I often liken to dirt and rock backcountry trails. Resilience pathways that go unused are like uneven, boulder-studded, winding trails that are hard to find and tricky to navigate.

The skills in this book will help you use your resilience pathways until they become smooth, easy to find, and readily available to enter.

Over time, and with regular use, your resilience pathways will be easy to find—with their own bright signs reading "Enter Here"—and easy to use. You can still imagine them as trails in the woods, if that is your thing. This is not a preference for urbanized over forested; it's about ease of entrance onto said route.

I'VE BEEN THERE TOO

Believe me when I say I've been there. This book comes sincerely from me in my darkest hours to you in yours. I really believe the tools in this book will help you. If they helped me...well, that's saying something, because I was *stressed*. Having a visceral reaction to stress is something I can remember as far back as age seven or eight. I was familiar with feeling my aching back when worries about my school performance mounted. I was also well aware of my pounding heart when bullies made me the target of their torments. I clearly remember the feeling of collapse in my chest when the dinner table conversations felt shaming, mocking, or mean.

As an adult, my tools for resilience from stress included my trusted go-tos of yoga and mindfulness meditation. These practices, which I used personally and taught professionally for over twenty years, helped alleviate a portion of my stress symptoms. I also found relief through insights I gained in periodic talk therapy. These were all helpful, until my stress level rose significantly. At a certain point, my stress level was so high that none of these trusted tools even made a dent in the solid steel of anxiety, physical pain, and stress activation I was suffering from.

Yes, my stress had been there in the background for years, but it wasn't something I had defined myself by. That is, until it began to define me. Over the course of a few particularly hard years, extreme-stress reactivity crept into more and more areas of my life. What precipitated all of this? In many ways, it was a perfect storm of events. But it was much more than the events themselves. At the heart of all of it was my body-mind system going totally off the rails, spinning out, and not having any idea about how to come back. As is the case for so many, my then-current extreme stress was not just a result of what was happening in my daily life. It was also the result of accumulated and unprocessed stress dating back decades.

So, yes, I did face a set of huge changes and challenges, prime real estate for stress imprints to move into. First, leaving a very established ten-year career and packing up to move to a totally new place where I was unknown and disoriented. Struggling with post-partum anxiety—which hit me like a ton of bricks, twice (a parting gift from each pregnancy). Then the amazingly complex task of learning to parent—this brought up *a lot* from my own childhood, which was not all roses and sunshine (really, far too little roses and sunshine). And then when I did return to the *traditional* workforce (I say traditional workforce because parenting at home *is work,* really—feeding, clothing, teaching, and otherwise nurturing small people is no trip to the spa!), I unfortunately took a job in an extremely toxic work environment where each day felt like I was throwing myself to the wolves—extremely ferocious and mean wolves—and that was absolutely the last straw! It all hugely caught me off guard. In a word, it was awful. With all that, and my already heavy load of more than forty years of stress residue and stress imprints, regular everyday normal stuff became so, so hard.

Living anxiously became my new normal. I got used to panic attacks at the grocery store and restaurants. Flop sweats at cocktail parties and while giving presentations at work. Sudden trembling and heart palpitations while just sitting at home, attempting to figure out how to manage my stress reactivity and anxiety. All these things, and more, happened regularly—and this was my body-mind's reaction to just normal daily life! I also limped my way through many stress-inducing things that were actually fairly run-of-the-mill stressors. Of course there were also peak stressful events, where my reactivity shot through the roof—a serious accident for each child (at separate times, thankfully), nearly losing our family's primary income during the great financial recession, the death of my father-in-law, to name just a few. When your normal life is putting you at an 8 (on a scale of 1 to 10) for stress-reactivity level, there isn't a lot higher to go when things truly get rough. In cases of actual emergency, panic attacks or total shutdown ensued. Full-bodied panic and overwhelm of the highest order, which sometimes was like a finger in an electric socket and sometimes completely disconnected me from myself and my life. Taken as a whole, my body-mind system had me dramatically, extraordinarily, shockingly afraid most of the time.

When I got to the point where anxiety accompanied me nearly everywhere, and high states of alarm happened every day, I had to find a way out. I was trying everything I could, from meditation and yoga to acupuncture, to talk therapy, to public speaking support groups, to herbs and dietary changes. Eventually I asked my physician if I had some rare disease that could explain all of the things that were happening to me. Happening *in me*. I even found myself hoping the answer was yes. A fantasized explanation of a disease felt more relieving than the truth—that chronic anxiety and overwhelm were running my life.

The battery of tests I underwent showed (ironically, to my disappointment) that I was healthy except for the extreme sweating, racing heart, dry mouth, insomnia, stomachaches, a.k.a. general panic that erupted in me when I was stressed, or nervous, or caught by surprise, or pressured, or, or, or...

I looked for answers and help everywhere I could. After *so* much seeking, and so much trying through meditating, talk therapy-ing, remembering, rehashing, willing, and general bargaining with some overseeing power somewhere, I found no relief, just the same persistent symptoms. On my doctor's recommendation, I even attempted to tranquilize myself with a prescription for Ativan, which just made me sloshy *and* stressed. "Ahh!" I thought. "You call this healthy?!" Splotches, trembling, insomnia, sweating, bellyaches, and the very palpable physical pain of being terrified most of the time? Well, I didn't call that healthy. I still don't.

Not only was my stress making my feel ill (and crazy), but these stress symptoms, like sweating and splotching, were really getting in the way of my daily life. It's hard to do your job, take care of your kids, or even just run errands when you're lit up like a Christmas tree and scared half to death of...you're not quite sure what. People regularly looked at me like "Whaaat is going on with you?!" And I didn't blame them; I was wondering the same thing. Living this way was, as you might imagine, intolerable. And maddeningly, I could not find methods, approaches, or practitioners that were helping.

It seemed to me that I should be able to get through this with the tools I already knew. I had spent a decade practicing and teaching yoga and helping clients and myself use yoga therapeutically. After seeing, and living, the limitations of yoga, I dedicated a decade to practicing and teaching mindfulness therapeutically. Using mindfulness therapeutically also fell short when serious stress, anxiety, and overwhelm became involved. I felt frustrated and misled. These highly, extensively recommended tools were not making a dent in my crisis.

Luckily, a few trails of crumbs led me in a new direction. I found a field that I believed would take me beyond the limits I had encountered with yoga and mindfulness, and I began graduate studies in mind-body medicine. Simultaneously, my persistent stress and anxiety brought me into my first somatic therapy sessions, and the inextricable connections between mind stress and body stress began to come into very clear focus.

In grad school, I promptly started researching lasting relief from stress and anxiety. The studies I found in the stacks led me to approaches and skills that I'd never heard of before. Researchers were writing about what I was living. These scientists explained that if we suffer from extreme stress it will show up in our body, not just our mind, and we cannot exclusively think and talk our way out of it; we must also *feel* our way through it.

Each week, I pored over research studies and emerging theories, gathering information and tools about people who had been where I was and had found some relief. And I also met with my skilled and patient somatic therapist—who, I was comforted to know, had been there herself and had found some relief. With my studies in the research stacks and on the couch, I was feeling incrementally relieved by this body-mind approach.

My graduate research and somatic therapy helped me to understand *viscerally* what was happening when the stress reaction was taking hold, and to experience *viscerally* what I could do about it. I learned how to decrease my reactivity from *within my body, physically* soothe my system, and, little by little, *feel* okay again (a good part of the time, that is). With my new somatic skills, I developed something that had been sorely lacking in my body-mind system: stress resilience. And this is what I want to share with you.

Explore This: How does stress feel in your body?

Assign a number from 1 to 10 to each bodily reaction
1 being very little, 10 being to an extreme

Heart pounding 1 2 3 4 5 6 7 8 9 10	Trembling 1 2 3 4 5 6 7 8 9 10	Sweating 1 2 3 4 5 6 7 8 9 10
Bracing 1 2 3 4 5 6 7 8 9 10	Clenching 1 2 3 4 5 6 7 8 9 10	Tingling 1 2 3 4 5 6 7 8 9 10
Body heat 1 2 3 4 5 6 7 8 9 10	Restlessness 1 2 3 4 5 6 7 8 9 10	Stomachache 1 2 3 4 5 6 7 8 9 10
Chest pain 1 2 3 4 5 6 7 8 9 10	Cold limbs 1 2 3 4 5 6 7 8 9 10	Numbness 1 2 3 4 5 6 7 8 9 10
Gut pain 1 2 3 4 5 6 7 8 9 10	Other _____ 1 2 3 4 5 6 7 8 9 10	Other _____ 1 2 3 4 5 6 7 8 9 10

RESEARCH-SUPPORTED APPROACH

This book is not based on a hunch or a guess. This book is based on solid data, dependable research studies, expert recommendations, current best practices, and my own research using the mind-body protocol you will find in the skills chapters. I call the protocol I developed the mind-body reset (MBR) approach. I chose this name because MBR can actually *reset* your baseline. Baseline is how you feel at rest, which for people *not* stuck on the stress autobahn is…restful. (If you find yourself thinking "Restful? What is that?" —read on!)

The MBR approach strengthens your ability to recover from stress and has been proven to increase resilience. The sensations you identified in the previous exercise will lessen as you use the tools in this book. Each tool you will learn is backed up with current scientific research and explanations of how and why it works. If, like me, you love the research, you'll have fun with these sections. If you prefer to directly dive into the tools, that's great too. It is the actual experience of these tools that will have the most dramatic effect on your stress reactivity. So read the research and then dive into the exercises, or go directly to the exercises and skip the research, but don't skip the exercises. If your body doesn't *experience* its own resilience, not much will shift, no matter how great your intellectual understanding of the science is. (Trust me, I've tried.)

Each time we travel on the roadways of resilience, related physiological and neurological pathways become *more* established and interconnected within our entire resilience network. As we use our stress highways less, they become *less* established and less connected within our stress networks. No need to hire a road crew; the woman- or man-power you need is right here, within your mind-body system.

After scouring the research literature and studying with cutting-edge experts, it is my privilege to share with you an embodied approach to wellness. The evidence-based tools in this book help us all to work with our evolutionary dispositions and our current dilemmas of feeling stuck in states of stress, overwhelm, and anxiety. The pathways of stress reactivity have become so well worn that overwhelm and anxiety are just the easiest paths for our mind-body system to choose. The tools in chapters 4 through 7 will help reroute you away from stress reactivity and instead toward stress resilience and stress recovery. There is also a host of materials available for download at the website for this book: http://www.newharbinger.com/44277. (See the very back of this book for more details.) With the tools of MBR, we can mitigate the stress in our *whole* mind-body system, not just one or the other.

INTO THE BODY

It may seem obvious to you, my fellow stress sufferer, that we experience stress *in our body* as well as our mind. But I had not been hearing that in my extensive searches for relief. Here's the big news: if we truly want relief from our stress, we have to resolve it *in the body* as well as the mind. Experts like Peter Levine, Bessel van der Kolk, Stephen Porges, and Robert Sapolsky insist that we must not rely on our heads alone.

In brief, Levine developed and trademarked the groundbreaking Somatic Experiencing therapeutic approach, taught and practiced all over the world; he has authored more than ten books on somatic regulation, and he continues to bring best practices for trauma and stress resolution into therapeutic communities. Van der Kolk founded the Trauma Center in Massachusetts, has authored more than 150 research articles on trauma and somatic regulation, and wrote the best-selling *The Body Keeps the Score: Brain, Mind, and Body in the Treatment of Trauma* (2014). Porges developed the pioneering polyvagal theory, which supports how our body and mind are inextricably linked for the pursuit of regulation; he has authored dozens of research articles on regulation and is a distinguished university scientist at Indiana University. Sapolsky, a professor at Stanford University, has authored numerous research articles and several books, including *Why Zebras Don't Get Ulcers* (2004)—which helped define how stress affects our entire body-mind system and leads to illness—and he is a research associate in Kenya. (Whoa, those are some impressive folks!)

These scientists' and educators' amazing works are the foundation of the science I will share with you throughout this book. Their research shows that when stress levels are exceptionally high, we need tools beyond what our mind can offer. In the following chapters, I'll unpack this further. I will highlight how the body is a more effective doorway than the mind to enter our stress-resilience pathways. In fact, in states of high stress, we need to move beyond the limits of thinking our way through it, and instead emphasize the other 97 percent of us that exists below the neck: our body.

WHAT IS A SOMATIC APPROACH?

A somatic approach uses the wisdom of your body, primarily, with your mind playing a secondary role. We'll use this somatic approach to recover from our bodies' enactment of stress, anxiety, and overwhelm. This is the foundation of the MBR tools. As I've said, we don't just *think* stress and anxiety; we also *feel* it. Our heart, lungs, and gut are unconsciously communicating to our arms, legs, eyes, and ears regularly throughout each day. It's all part of an intricate system designed to assess danger and protect us from harm before we even begin to think through the whole situation. It's doing its thing even when you are not paying any attention or thinking about it in the slightest. This is your nervous system, and this amazing system will be unpacked much more in the next chapter.

When your body registers safety, this system is a well-run factory, a happy place, an environment of contentment. Your chest will likely feel relaxed or open. Breathing is easy and breaths are full. Belly happily does its job, digesting, extracting nutrients, and comfortably eliminating. What's more, eyes function well and accurately see the surroundings; mouth is comfortably moist, and food tastes good; body temperature is even and comfortable, adjusting appropriately to the current environment; muscles are relaxed, engaged only as much as the task demands. In a word, when this system assesses safety, you feel *good*.

Hyperactivation

When the body registers threat, this system goes right in as a first responder. The factories just mentioned all shut down or shift modes, as the body attempts to instantly transform into a lean, mean fighting machine. We start to breathe erratically, often quickly and shallowly (light-headed sometimes?); we evacuate or lock down our bowels (diarrhea or constipation, anyone?); our mouth goes dry (sudden thirst?); sweat pools under our arms, or hands, or back (wet marks?); maybe we clench our jaw, contract our neck, squeeze our shoulders, butt, or thighs (chronic pain?). We begin the adrenaline rollercoaster ride. These reactions are part of our survival system's fight-or-flight mode. It can also be described as a state of hyperactivation. Activation is turning the system on to be engaged and at the ready. Fight-or-flight mode is: *A. Lot. Of. Ready.*

Hypoactivation

And of course, what goes up must come down, and we can find ourselves on a long bender of being either all on, some version of flight-or-flight, or all off, some version of freeze or shutdown. Freeze or shutdown reverses the processes just described: we breathe too slowly or infrequently; we go cold, not producing enough body heat; our muscles slacken, with insufficient energy or effort. Freeze or shutdown is a slippery response. On the one hand, it can be marked by feeling disconnected, spaced-out, unable to follow what is happening around you, lethargic, numb, apathetic. This is called *hypoactivation*. Not enough get-up-and-go; hardly enough to just get through the day. However, it can also entail all the activation and readiness described for hyperactivation (pounding heart, muscle tension, vigilant scanning), just held very captive under a stillness that is anything but calm. In many cases of hypoactivation, *hyper*activation is living right beneath the surface of the statue-like state. Freeze and shutdown are coping mechanisms that the body naturally initiates when the stress we face is too overwhelming or too persistent, or happens too quickly for us to process in any other way. We can draw a simplified distinction between freeze and shutdown: freeze = not ready; shutdown = not here.

Explore This: Do I tend toward hyper- or hypoactivation?

Circle the reactivity you feel familiar with in each column. Then total your score for each side.

Hyperactivation	Hypoactivation
Speedy	Frozen
Aggressive	Passive
Restless	Lethargic
Quick-fire and reactive	Slow and withdrawn
Piercingly hyperfocused	Unable to focus
Sweating	Numb or cold
Total Score	**Total Score**

Do you see a higher score for either hyper- or hypoactivation? Or are you fairly equal with the two modes of response? Knowing your symptoms of activation and your tendencies toward either hyper- or hypo- can help you recognize when stress activation is occurring in your body. And recognition of activation is the first step to soothing the activation.

ANOTHER OPTION

Riding the peaks and valleys of hyper- and hypoactivation, we rarely get to enjoy the middle ground *between* all and nothing. A somatic approach can teach our automatic body response that there are actually other options, not just those of hyper- and hypo- activation. We probably know well that we have a great capacity for hyperactivation, the flight/flight mode, and hypoactivation, the freeze/shutdown response. However, we also have a range of responses between these two extremes, a mode of *functional* activation. Like the tale of Goldilocks, this functional activation is based on the not too much and not too little model. With somatic regulation, we find a range of activation that our mind-body systems finds to be just right.

FUNCTIONAL ACTIVATION

Activation is not a bad thing; activation is also known as engagement. Levine explains that a return to functional activation returns us to our basic aliveness, goodness, and power. Functional activation is a state in which we feel able to show up; we become attentive and available. It's an aware yet calm state. With functional activation, you are *engaged, present, ready.*

Because functional activation is an embodied state, as opposed to a purely mental state, a somatic approach enlists the body in the process of finding, returning to, and building the capacity for functional activation. With somatic regulation, we teach the body how to access this state largely on its own. In day-to-day life, we can't continuously think through a checklist in order to be engaged, present, and ready. In a state of functional activation, we access our alert yet calm awareness from an embodied state built on a *felt sense* of presence, safety, and ease.

With somatic regulation on board, we don't need to try to think our way through slowing our heart rate, easing our digestion, or lessening our sweat production. These functions are not usually very successfully governed by thoughts anyway. These are jobs of the body. We have evolved for millions of years to have a fine-tuned automatic response within our body. So with somatic regulation, we are working in harmony with evolution. We use the body to heal the body. In this process, the whole mind-body resets from a baseline of stress and overwhelm to a baseline of alert and calm. And at the center of our experience we feel here, safe, and okay.

WHAT IS SELF-REGULATION?

Self-regulation is the process of skillfully moving between these three states and of recovering from extreme states when necessary. We all move into hyper- or hypoactivation at times. At times, we need these extreme states. It's the *habit* of going to these states as our first response, the ensuing habitual reliance on these states, and getting stuck in these states that is the challenge addressed in this book. Hyper- and hypoactivation can become such well-worn pathways in our system that we begin to regularly use these emergency states as daily functioning systems. I probably don't have to tell you that having breakfast, going to work, seeing friends, or answering text messages from a state of emergency is no way to live.

Self-regulation is the ability to use our body and brain to come back from hyper- and hypoactivation states. Reclaiming our ability to self-regulate liberates us from living life as if danger is lurking around every corner. Our mind-body system recovers its flexibility, health, and ability to deal with stress and the like. Self-regulation is a skill many of us need to learn. This book teaches that skill through the doorway of the body.

Flexible Reactivity

A healthy mind-body system can *appropriately* move into states of *necessary* reactivity and then move out again. We are not aiming for a constant state of being chilled out; that is not what life always calls for. If I'm standing on a sidewalk, about to step onto the street, when I realize that a huge truck is barreling down the road toward my intersection, I want to instantly move into hyperactivation or flight mode and get out of the way. I *want* a surge of adrenaline; my heart rate to rapidly increase; body temperature to rise; increased muscle tension in my legs; narrowing of my scope of vision to the truck; hearing only relevant information about getting out of the way. This is all called for, appropriate, necessary. Yay, well-functioning nervous system! It took care of *automatically* reacting, bringing me appropriately into a state of hyperactivation. Who has time to think through a checklist when your life is in danger?

If, however, we do not recover from this event and we get stuck in hyperactivation, we can go from the street-crossing incident into our first meeting of the day, still on very high alert, still in hyperactivation. We might shout at a colleague who questions our proposal, or nearly jump through the roof when we hear our phone ring.

If our system cannot sustain high alert, often due to exhaustion from overuse or overwhelm, we might move into a state of hypoactivation. In this instance, we may manage to get out of the way of the truck, but the whole incident occurs as if in a dream. Then we go on to the next task of the day in a state of disconnection. We hardly notice a friend speaking to us, and we forget to send the three important emails we had been enthusiastically working on the day before.

Inflexible Reactivity

Inflexible reactivity is persistently heading straight into states of intense stress reactivity, no matter the situation. If you have found yourself walking into a room full of strangers, boarding an airplane, heading off to work, or going on a date, and so on, while having an automatic reaction similar to that of nearly being hit by a truck, the upcoming mind-body tools are for you. Inflexible reactivity is also getting stuck in your stress reactivity instead of being able to return to functional activation once the stress has passed. If you were to be nearly hit by a car (in actuality, a driver just cut into your lane aggressively) and you were to find yourself flinching at every sudden movement that whole morning or growling at each conversation you have that afternoon, you would be stuck in reactivity. Flexibility is possible, but after enduring extreme or prolonged stress, our systems need a little help remembering those resilience routes.

Stress Triggers

Simply put, a stress trigger is the stuff in your life that sends your system into hyper- or hypoactivation, fight/flight and freeze/shutdown, respectively. When faced with a stress trigger, your mind-body system may have become habituated to stress reactivity. As I mentioned before, your body might be exceedingly good at stress reactivity. This can play out as hyper- and hyporeactivity in many different situations. Maybe you go into fight/flight or freeze/shutdown mode when you're running late and are caught in traffic; when you're being evaluated by a supervisor at work; during an argument with family members; parenting a less than cooperative child; or facing sudden change, like illness or loss.

There is a wide range of symptoms. Stress reactivity comes in all shapes and sizes and can show up in many areas of your life. Knowing your triggers and the way your system responds to stress is important. If you do not see your symptoms described here, I encourage you to add your own experience to the descriptions as you read through this book. Gaining the skills of recovering from stress triggers is what the MBR offers. We couldn't do away with *all* life triggers, even if we tried, so here we learn how to recover from them (and maybe, we'll also offload a few of the really unnecessary triggers along the way).

Try This: Notice Your Stress Triggers

Over the next week or two, take notice of what your stress triggers might be. See if certain types of situations repeatedly bring about stress reactivity. Situations that consistently elicit stress reactivity could be stress triggers for you.

No need to understand why. Just explore the patterns.

It's helpful to identify when you are experiencing stress sensations and take note of what is occurring at that time. Is it loud where you are? Are things hectic? Do you feel alone? Is there pressure? Is your time too unstructured? Do you feel unseen? You may notice, for example, that each time you have to give some kind of presentation you feel hyperactivation. You might find that when you are navigating to a new destination, you feel hypoactivation.

If you've identified a tendency toward hyper- or hypoactivation, you can look for signs of either of those dispositions. You can also consult the sensation chart you responded to earlier as a reminder of what kinds of sensations tend to accompany stress for you.

This may take some practice. It's common to be unaware of our stress. Mild dissociation from your stress is thousands of years of evolution playing out in you. Bringing gentle curiosity to your stress triggers will be important. We don't want to stress ourselves out about being stressed. Can you kindly and supportively learn more about your triggers this week?

After each time you notice a trigger, it will be helpful to your resilience to take a few moments to *return from* the trigger. Going through the steps from exercise 1, feeling your body settle, noticing sensations of softening and support wherever you are—all of these can help for now. In later chapters, you'll gain several more tools for *returning* from stress.

BODY AND MIND IN CONCERT

As Bessel van der Kolk wrote, the body keeps the score. Our body records and remembers stress reactions viscerally, while our mind tells the story through words and mental pictures. I think of the body memories as being like a child in class raising their hand for help. With hand in the air, the child calls out, "Is it my turn to get some support and resolution?" This is what the body symptoms are asking.

As you work through this book you will think about, maybe write about, or perhaps talk about your stressful events and memories. Then you will use the skills outlined here to call on that memory with its hand raised and help to soothe it. We'll use language, because that is how we communicate, but we will also circle back repeatedly to the body, and the unspoken messages it is communicating to us. The body is remembering, below the surface, waiting for an opportunity to repair what has been injured.

CALLED TO ACTION

As I began to feel better and better in my own life—regulated, flexible within my nervous system, and more often okay than not okay—I kept wondering, why are the skills and approaches for mind *and* body stress recovery so difficult to find? As the relief really started to sink into my own body, I wanted to shout from the rooftops. I yearned to call out, "Everyone who is living with the deep pain of anxiety and extreme stress needs to hear about these incredibly relieving tools! You don't have to keep suffering from your painful symptoms. You don't have to just get by anymore. You can really live!"

This book is my proverbial shout from the rooftops. All of us know how to get into states of stress reactivity; evolutionary instincts take over and lead the way. The skills we need to develop now, in this day and age, are how to get back out of these well-worn stress reaction pathways. Mind *and* body regulation offers incredible tools for getting *back out* of stress, anxiety, and overwhelm. Not just in your head, but in your body too. Welcome to your recovery. Ease awaits you.

CHAPTER 2

Possible Pitfalls for Stress Resilience

Unfortunately, not every therapeutic approach out there helps you *feel* internal okayness. Those that rely too heavily on the (busy) mind might interrupt your progress. For a felt sense of well-being and safety, approaches that keep you distanced from your body and way too up in your head are a good place *not* to start. When we are stuck upstairs, our embodied smarts can be undermined. It's hard to hear our body intelligence over the soundtrack of our relentless yackety-yak mind. Choruses of coulda, woulda, shoulda are not exactly finger-tapping fun. When we try to *think* our way into *feeling* better, the busy mind takes us toward stress instead of away from it.

OH, THE BUSY MIND

When we're in a state of stress, the yackety-yak is not just annoying background noise; the tales our stress brain spins can be truly horrific. As the introspective and candid author Anne Lamott has said, "My mind is like a bad neighborhood I try not to go into alone." So let's not go in alone. If you take along your body, you are not alone in your mind; you have the other 97 percent of you there too!

Let's take a bird's-eye look at what to avoid in the neighborhoods of the head and then navigate into some of the safe districts of the body.

THE STUFF THAT'S HARD TO TALK ABOUT

On my search for relief from my extreme stress and anxiety, I ran into some very unexpected

> When stress is extreme, you *feel* your stress and anxiety in your body, not just *think* it in your head.

roadblocks. These roadblocks were initially a poor choice for me because of their heady nature, but with my extreme stress, they quickly became a real problem for my body too. These are the kind of blockades you're not exactly excited to talk about, because they don't—at first glance—seem to be blocking anyone else. When relief is elusive, the "What's wrong with me?" questions often start popping up. It was this "What's wrong with me?" question that led me to look further. But to answer the question honestly, I had to be brave, and to be willing to say that some approaches that seemed...so well respected, highly recommended, and popular...were not helping *me*. And when I started to share this, I realized I wasn't alone. Funny that this would even be hard to name. When I am totally clearheaded I know, of course we are all unique, of course we all need to carefully select the approaches that work best for us as individuals. Even so, I needed encouragement. And I found it with researcher and author Brené Brown.

"We can talk about courage, love, and compassion until we sound like a greeting card store, but unless we are willing to have an honest conversation about what gets in the way, we will never change, never ever" Brené Brown (2010) said to me emphatically (through my headset, via her audiobook) while I was in the midst of my research. Her words shone a light on what I was finding in myself, colleagues, clients, *and* the scientific literature. The data kept revealing that there are many ways a nervous system can get stuck on a kind of autopilot and drive us directly *back to* the land of stress, anxiety, and overwhelm; the very place we're trying *not* to hang out in. It turns out that choosing your unique healing routes for your unique system is really important and takes self-awareness, self-compassion, and maybe even bravery.

NOT EVERY TOOL IS RIGHT FOR EVERY JOB

You wouldn't pick up a plunger if you really needed a hammer. Choosing tools can be complex; some tools are loud, some quiet; some excavate like bulldozers, some like a hand trowel; some approaches move quickly and intensely, some take a slow and gentle approach. With extreme stress imprints, less is more, and more is...too much.

"Less" is any approach that soothes the system; it's easy does it. "More" is any approach that consistently agitates the system; that feels abrasive, volatile, or severe; that's got the potential to blow things up. There are many approaches that can take us into our stress too fast, or too deeply, or too often—and experiences that are too fast or deep, or happen too often, even supposedly helpful ones, easily masquerade as stressors themselves. If the tool *creates* stress, it might not be the best tool. While I could focus on many different tools or methods of stress reduction that have the potential to be too much, in the following sections, I'll just mention two common and widely recommended approaches: mindfulness meditation (MM) and exposure emphasis (EE) talk therapy.

Healing approaches often emphasize, or are driven by, either your mind or your body. The emphasis is like the motor of a train locomoting it in the right or wrong direction. When it comes to extreme stress, thought-driven approaches often don't end up at the destinations of self-regulation and functional activation—there's too much background noise distracting and agitating along the way. In contrast, body-driven trains *do* often take us to the desti-

> Experiences that happen too fast, are too deep, or are repeated too often can become stressors themselves—even if they are meant to be healing experiences.

nations of recovery—which I'll discuss more in chapter 3. This is a big part of why MM and EE therapies might be two potential hazards to avoid on your path to healing.

Ironically, I entered graduate school to pursue a deeper understanding of how mindfulness and meditation could lessen anxiety and extreme stress. Yet the more I saw the data in the research literature, the more I had to shift from a mindfulness focus to a "bodyfulness" focus. Current science continues to show that body-based methods, not head-based methods, are our best tools for extreme-stress recovery.

Honestly, I was as surprised as anyone that the tools I had once relied on were no longer helping. Mindfulness had been a go-to for me for years. I had been a mindfulness meditator for more than fifteen years and had been teaching it to groups and individuals for more than eight years. I was teaching at one of the most renowned meditation centers in the world, Spirit Rock, when the practice of meditation started to back-fire on me, significantly. When my stress and overwhelm became extreme, sitting with and watching my experience was not soothing, as it had once been. In fact, I was literally witnessing myself melting down, day after day, meditation after meditation, and this was steadily making things much much worse. This certainly isn't the case for everyone, but as I've come to find, it is the case for enough of us to warrant a little explanation in this book, as follows.

PROGRESS MAY BE INTERRUPTED

Everything concerning mindfulness that I had read and studied up to that point promised that it was a reliable tool for stress and anxiety relief. All the mindfulness writings and teaching I encountered suggested that I just needed to be patient, detach more, and allow my experience to be as it was. The wisest of teachers were indicating that this approach would eventually help lessen my anxiety and overwhelm. As this kept failing, I was becoming more and more lost. I kept wondering why my symptoms were getting increasingly worse with each of my earnest attempts to relieve them.

Meanwhile, I sought therapy to help with my extreme stress levels. Each week, in a technique based on exposure to one's stresses, I would tell and retell the stress from my childhood, the stress in my current life, and the stress I feared lay ahead for me. And as you might guess, I felt *more* stressed! While our minds may love to ceaselessly dwell on any number of painful episodes we've lived through, as far as our body acti-vation is concerned, the dwelling can make things sticky. And these sticky sensations can glue themselves to our stress-centric survival brain, making it feel like it is all happening again and again…and again.

One definition of patience I read called it "suffering without com-plaint." Yup, that's what I was doing. Until I did start to complain, and then to speculate: am I the only one who is having this experience? Are other people suffering without complaint as their symptoms of stress and anxiety *increase* under the gaze of mindful awareness and exposure therapy? At first, I asked—quietly—if fellow meditators and friends in exposure therapy were have any similar experiences. Then I started surveying—tentatively, cautiously—other mindfulness teachers and discussing my experiences with exposure therapy educators. This led me to scour the research literature to find out what's going on with mindfulness, exposure therapy, and extreme stress. Now I say—out loud—that we noncomplaining sufferers are not alone. This was more common than I thought, and certainly much more prevalent than was being talked or written about in the news and media with the current mindfulness craze and exposure therapy as a gold standard treatment for trauma.

It turns out, repeatedly dunking in the too-deep waters of stress doesn't work so well for many of us; it just feels like nearly drowning all over again. This is a hugely important point for somatic healing—easy does it, less is more. Without the addition of a buoy, raft, or tug line, immersing in the waters of suffering alarms our body-mind system. Sufferers of extreme stress need to take lots of breaks to breathe, rest, and find momentary "islands of safety," a particularly lovely phrase from Levine (1997). The somatic skills in this book will offer you just such islands. Time and space to catch your breath, rest your tired bones, and feel some relief. And that resilience and relief is a *felt experience* facilitated by your amazing nervous system.

Remember two things:

- When *processing* extreme stress, too much is too much.

- To increase stress *regulation*, less can be more.

Meditating or being with intense stress memories for extended periods can *increase* your felt stress. Diving deeply into describing stress events can *overexpose* your mind-body to the felt memory.

Try This: Seeing What's Okay

Read through these instructions completely, then try out this exercise, referring back to the instructions as needed.

Take a moment to simply look around. Can you see something in your environment or out a window that you enjoy seeing or find pleasing in some way? Scan your surroundings for something. Perhaps a view of a tree, a painting on a wall, a lovely quality of light. What you choose is not important; letting your *eyes rest* on it is important. Allow your eyes to just take this image in; perhaps your focus even softens a bit. Let your eyes do what they may; take your time, there is no rush.

Can you now let your breath deepen? Invite slightly longer breaths in, and slightly longer breaths out. Repeat this a few times.

Last, feel your body in this moment. Can you sense any ease, even just a bit? Notice any part of you that feels okay, or even simply neutral. Just try this for a moment or two; no need to stay here any longer than you feel like. Easy does it. Less can be more.

You'll find audio recordings for this and the other exercises in this book available for download at http://www.newharbinger.com/44277.

YOUR AMAZING NERVOUS SYSTEM

Especially if you have suffered a great deal of extreme stress or trauma, your amazing nervous system might do well with some tools and clearly *not* do well with others. Your system may be quite sensitive; listen to those sensitivities, as they are very important for somatically based healing.

We each have a hub—a sensitivities hub, if you will—inside of us, functioning around the clock. This hub always keeps tabs on what is going on—how sensitized we are to whatever it is, and how we need to prepare for what the events may be. Twenty-four hours a day, this hub is checking out the goings on outside and inside of us to be sure everything is okay, or at least *okay enough.*

After determining okay enough or not okay enough, this hub is your epicenter for reactivity, reacting and adapting with lightning speed and robust force. If all is well, this epicenter gracefully downshifts you and you'll cruise along feeling safe, physically comfortable, and clear thinking. If all is *not well*, there is a quick shifting of gears and a nearly instantaneous acceleration into "get it done" mode, pushing the gas pedal as far as needed to reach the goal. And of course, with that kind of speed, our safety, comfort, and mental functioning fly out the window, for all of us. We're just wired this way. The too much, too fast, too deep I mentioned before drags our nervous system directly away from safe, comfortable, and clear thinking.

YOUR NERVOUS SYSTEM ON AUTOPILOT

Ongoing "get it done" mode can create stress autopilot, or stress-a-lot, as one might say. If stress is a frequent guest for you, a "skill" for your hub can be: accelerate first and think about it later. For those of us who have lived through periods of extreme stress, anxiety, and overwhelm, this hub can get stuck in its "things are *not* okay enough" position. When you're stuck in *not* okay, this center is less like a corral of okayness and more like the OK corral—quick-fire and passionate in its reactivity, while menacingly looking for trouble.

Once not okay has happened in a big way for you, either repeated too often or occurring in a whopping all-at-once stressor, "not okay" is no longer just a guest; it becomes a needy roommate, always nagging you to do what it says. Not okay becomes what your system does best—and onto the stress autobahn you go. Your system becomes very good at extreme reactivity—and remember, your well-oiled machine of reactivity loves the familiar. Even when you've exhausted nearly all your inner strength and feel like you're on your last legs, the system usually chooses familiar over all else. (The old adage that how you do anything is how you do everything applies here.) How your system has been accustomed to reacting is how it will continue to react. If stress-a-lot has been your go-to, your system will go to it. Pedal to the metal, full steam ahead...

But hey, this system is just trying to help us out. It is committed to keeping us at the ready for whatever is coming our way. Except...with quick-fire reactivity and trouble-scanning, something that one might assume would be in the okay column, like going to a party, can *feel* like something squarely in the not-okay column—being surrounded by wolves, for example. Likewise, a job interview can prompt the same reaction as a high-speed car chase. Or life stressors like amassed debt can trigger sensations of being in a room with too little air. As Robert Sapolsky, Stanford professor and researcher, points out (2004), this hub's accelerator response is so consistent and robust that humans have been shown to have nearly the same physical reaction to being afraid while speaking publicly as they would to being harassed on a darkened street. That's some stress autopilot—stress-a-lot!

Explore This: Does your system have an autopilot?

Read over these common stress reactions and identify any that are frequent visitors for you.

(This is a very partial list; please use the blank spaces to fill in *your* unique responses to stress.)

What Does Your System Do on Autopilot?	
In my body	In my mind
hot flashes	racing thoughts
nausea	worry
headache	anger
coldness	negativity
numbness	fixation
sweating	spaciness
trembling	hypervigilance
constipation	sadness
aching back or neck	rapid-fire problem solving
feeling far away	inability to think
other _____	other _____
other _____	other _____

Your Body Is Your Pilot

This hub, a.k.a. your central nervous system, I like to call "okay-central" because its ultimate job is to keep us okay—homeostasis and all that jazz. Okay-central is all about the body; your body is its pilot. This body-centric system spans from your lower skull to the base of your torso. It starts at your instinctive primitive brain, which governs *body* instincts; runs down your brainstem, which is where your brain remembers *sensations,* not sonnets; winds through your neck; and has many satellite survey centers sprinkled throughout your chest, belly, gut, and reproductive organs, where it culminates in the bowl of your pelvis. Body. Body. Body!

Okay-central governs your heart rate, blood pressure, and breathing depth. These alone have a huge effect on how okay, or not, you feel; it's hard to feel at ease while gasping for air with a pounding heart. (Sound familiar?) This hub also runs your body temperature and sweat production, a significant contribution to our felt sense of safety—we can be so scared we sweat bullets, or so overwhelmed we're as cold as ice. (Careful wardrobe planning a norm for you?) Okay-central is also in charge of digestion and elimination. (Gut tied in knots over meetings at work? Get the runs or blocked up every time you're confronted by you-know-who?) Also, this center plays a huge role in brain functioning. The balance or lack thereof in our okay-central dictates whether or not we can think clearly. When the nonverbal primitive brain of our central nervous system is running the show, it's lights out in the reasoning, empathy, and complex thought centers of our evolved front brain. (Ever been caught suddenly unable to access even the most basic words—in your native language, no less?)

Body Takes You to Not-So-Nice and Nice Places to Be

When there's a knot in the pit of your stomach, and/or your heart is racing, and/or the hair on the back of your neck is standing on end, and/or sweat is trickling down your sides, your nervous system is ramping up. This is the fear response. In it you'll feel ill-at-ease and distrustful and have lightning-speed reactivity. When this kind of activation takes hold, your entire body begins preparations to save you! And okay-central will determine things are *not* okay. Next, your system will lean toward either flight-or-fight mode (hyperreactivity) or freeze-or-shutdown mode (hyporeactivity). Flight or fight involves running away to safety or fighting for your life, respectively.

Freeze or shutdown will render you stiff and speechless or cause significant functions of your body-brain to shutdown, respectively. You freeze or shutdown if your system deems the active options of flight or fight impossible because the threat seemed insurmountable.

We have evolved to do these things—flee, fight, freeze, or shutdown—for good reasons. And these can be adaptive, brilliant, necessary reactions to a serious and imminent threat. Your evolutionary smarts will be covered more in future chapters. But! In the event that you are *not* facing a major threat—maybe you are merely stuck in traffic, giving a presentation, paying overdue bills, or in conflict with a mate—this kind of reactivity is no longer an aid. Evolution is no longer coming to the rescue. These instincts and automatic reactivity can become a serious burden. That burden is *dysregulation*. This is a not-so-nice destination.

Fear not! There is a whole range of functionality between do or die. The between mode of *regulation*, better described as a process, an experience. This body-led process is largely a felt experience—although it does also engender clear thinking (nice perk!). Regulation is *sensing* safety, *embodying* presence, *being* at ease, and dadada da da da da, *feeling* groovy. This is most definitely a nice destination.

The territory of regulation includes many different landscapes that share these common elements: situationally appropriate responses, rather than a racing heart in a grocery store or sweating bullets on an airplane; the felt sense of okayness, rather than feeling alone, annoyed, or attacked; and access to high-level thoughts—"Ahhh, it wasn't age-related cognitive decline after all!" With the tools of somatic regulation, we'll hang out in this terrain of groovy. We'll get to know the many streams, valleys, and peaks of these lands, through our *direct felt experience*. And of course, we'll uncover how to navigate *back to* these places after being pulled away—which we all are, regularly. Small detours are to be expected; driving headlong into trouble again and again…maybe let's not. (Opting for nice instead of not-so-nice here, people.)

BUT EVERYONE IS DOING IT

With all this hair-trigger reactivity in our system, we really do need to proceed with caution as we embark on our own healing journey—a journey toward regulation and ease. There are many approaches that work well for moderate stressors but really aren't appropriate for extreme stressors. And just because it's part of the popular culture at this time doesn't necessarily qualify it for *your* journey. Any approach that takes you into your stress memories and stress sensations too quickly or intensely—and I do mean INTO, all caps, major dive—is questionable. Deep somatic healing requires that, with care and attentiveness, you ask your body what approaches are best for you, instead of asking your head. You are your own laboratory, and your felt experience is your very best guide when it comes to somatic regulation. Any methods that amplify your stress—for more than short and rescindable periods—should be suspect.

I've heard many people over the years trying to convince themselves that an unhelpful approach was indeed helpful. It is easy to think that the shaky, scared, or otherwise bad feeling you get when you do X is your own fault or shortcoming. It's very easy to blame yourself and to try even harder—and harder—to make some highly recommended approaches work for you. I felt compelled to understand this phenomenon. So I

> A felt sense of ease, well-being, and safety—all of these are paramount on the road to recovery from extreme stress; it's important that you are often in the company of these traveling mercies.

spent years researching this topic—I did this for both of us. Now I say with confidence, it's not you—or me! That uncomfortable feeling you got from that ill-fitting healing approach: the stomachache, or insomnia, or eczema, or general anxiety increase that lasted for days, or weeks, or months—is called reliving your stress.

Remember the automatic reactivity discussed earlier in this chapter? That's what that stomachache, insomnia, eczema, general anxiety, et cetera, was. And automaticity is, well, automatic—it just happens. It's the way we are wired. You do not have to go through that in order to heal. Take a look at these potential hazards for yourself, and see what the best navigation routes are for you.

CAREFULLY SELECTING THE TOOLS FOR YOUR TOOL KIT

The first step in careful selection is assessing and questioning the effectiveness of the tools you currently have in your kit. Is sitting with your stress right for you? I encourage you to take stock of your unique experiences *before, during,* and *after* sitting with your stress. Come to your own conclusions on whether it is helpful for you at this particular stage of your stress recovery. At times it may be just right, and at others it may be missing the mark. My friend and colleague Jose shared this reflection of a time he listened to his instincts as they told him intensive meditation was *not* the right tool for the job at that time.

When Jose was in his twenties, he set off for what would be a three-month-long silent meditation retreat. The first few days showed glimpses of what could be ahead for him. Some very scary and emotional memories from his past were popping up during the meditation sessions, and he was feeling that the hour-after-hour exposure to some of his difficult history might be too much for him at that time. After a few very painful days—emotionally and physically—he got the idea in his head that he didn't need meditation right then; what he really needed was to have a vacation and relax a bit, to be with friends and family. It was a very difficult decision, but he decided to leave the retreat. Initially, he doubted his pull toward days full of rest instead of the days full of intensive meditation he had intended for himself. However, he said that in hindsight, he thanks his lucky stars that his intuition spoke up and he listened. He explained that it would have been so normal for him to push himself to stay, even force himself to. Instead, he left what he feels was likely to be three months of full catastrophe. He got a taste of sitting with his stress and overwhelm during those first days at the retreat; he's glad he didn't stay for the main course. That wasn't the right time for him to do so. I'm guessing we've all been there, with part of us saying "This situation is definitely too much," while another part is trying to convince ourself that it will work if we just try harder. Luckily, Jose did not fall under the sway of his inner bully.

Sometimes, we ignore this inner guidance or gut feeling and cajole ourselves in a *seemingly* good direction. Or as Winnie the Pooh says, "It might have been a very good idea for a very different day." I've had meditation students tell me they felt afraid, jittery, or like ants were crawling all over them as they tried to sit and breathe with their experience. *Oh no*, I've thought. *Your body-mind system is trying to ask you to stop. There are gentler ways to help yourself besides forcing approaches that aren't soothing your system.* I'm glad to share that the "just keep sitting there" perspective is shifting, and not only is the tide turning, but researchers caution that no therapeutic approach should be expected to work for everyone.

Neuroscientist Katherine Kerr, who runs a research lab for mindfulness studies at Brown University, implores, "Don't believe the hype" (Heuman 2014). Kerr says that popular media are promoting "the idea that every person who has any mental abilities should be doing mindfulness meditation…I don't think the science supports that." Asked what kind of evidence she, as a scientist, would encourage people to consider when thinking of mindfulness as a therapeutic remedy, Kerr replied, "each person should consider his or her own concrete experiences. That should be central…we should ask *ourselves*, how did it make *me feel* while meditating and how did *I feel* later in the day?"

I fully agree. Let's refer to our own experiences, our *felt* experiences. If you're good at extreme reactivity, then it's all too easy for your system to head straight into it. Sitting and mindfully witnessing that intensity, or elaborating on those memories, or other [fill in the blank] too much, too fast, or too often may not be the best remedy for you. Your own experience of safety and ease must lead your way.

Try This: Inquire Within

Is this tool right for you at this time in your life, with the particulars of what you're facing?

How do you feel *before, during,* and *after* meditation?

Does meditating create some ease and settling for you? If yes, wonderful, add it to your kit.

Does meditating cause nervousness, restlessness, dissociation, anxiety, or stress? If yes, do not put it in your kit. This book has many other tools for you to work with.

In a 2014 research study, some participants of the study benefited from mindfulness; for others, mindfulness had a negative effect—same mindfulness practice, similar ailments going into the study, very different reactions to the tool within the group. Seventy-nine veterans suffering from stress, anxiety, chronic pain, and depression, volunteered to be taught MM via a nine-week mindfulness-based stress reduction (MBSR) course (Serpa, Taylor, and Tillisch 2014). For sitting meditation, participants were taught to pay attention to their breath and if thoughts came to mind, to notice the thoughts and then return their attention to their breath. These are very standard meditation instructions. The study results showed that only thirty-two out of seventy-nine participants experienced a decrease in emotional anxiety after the course completion. That leaves forty-six of the participants who did not experience any relief from anxiety. It is also significant that for three of the volunteers, their anxiety was *worse* after the course. Mindfulness appears not to be one size fits everyone.

Similar variations in helpful effects are being recognized with therapies that delve too quickly and too deeply into the client's stresses, traumas, and pain. In the article "The Limits of Talk" (Wylie 2004), Bessel van der Kolk notes that often his patients couldn't talk about their traumatic memories effectively and if he pushed them to try harder to talk things through, they began "hyperventilating, shaking, yelling, crying, became physically agitated, or just collapsed in a state of helpless fear and dread." In my own practice, I see similar outcomes. One client said to me, "I'm so glad I don't have to just tell you my story another time. I'm sick of telling my story, telling it makes me feel bad all over again." This is not a defect of some kind; telling one's stress stories all over again is shown *to be stressful,* and it can literally make us feel physically—biochemically—bad. This happens when retelling our story reactivates our stress memory, and leads to *reliving* the memory. It's not just a matter of comfort that we not push ourselves into shoes that don't fit; it's *central* to our stress resilience.

It's *not* all in your head; it's in your body too. We've got to get below the neck to deeply heal the somatic wounds left by struggle and stress.

And we've got to do this gently, reassuringly, and slowly or the body just gets sucked back into the struggle again.

In a study of adults with panic disorder and excessive fears, participants' reactions to exposure therapy were examined (Siegmund et al. 2011). A panic and fear group was compared to a healthy control group. The study used a flooding technique wherein the therapist boosted the participants' fear "as much as possible" by continuously directing the participants to fear-increasing thoughts, images, sensations, and so on. The therapist did this until each participant reached a fear level of 10 on a 1-to-10 scale.

The scientists found that the panic and fear group was significantly more afraid during this flooding technique than the healthy control group. They also found that, after flooding the participants on three separate occasions, the participants who remained afraid during each flooding session—meaning their fears did not decrease from session one to session three—did not benefit from the therapy. The exposure did not help them recover from fear; quite the reverse: it scared them. Overall, at the end of the study, after eight cognitive behavioral therapy sessions and three flooding exposures, the combined scores for the participants showed that participants still had 60 percent of the fear that they began with. A clear example of being thrown directly into the deep end, no line, no buoy. Our mind-body systems do not always thrive in circumstances like these.

Try This: Are your go-to tools working for you?

Explore your levels of activation before, during, and after you dive deeply into your stress memories.

Does this "get it all out" approach feel relieving? If yes, great! find a trusted listener and be heard.

If going too fast or too deeply creates more stress, perhaps try an easy-does-it approach. Less can be more. Share bite-sized pieces of your story with a trusted listener, then take a break and talk about something relieving. Or write out just the beginning of the stress event in your journal, being brief, then shift to jotting down things you are grateful for. Later, do the same thing with the middle of the stress event, briefly writing it down, followed by gratitude or doodling or a cup of tea. Then the same with the end of the stress event: a brief description of the ending. Be sure to take a break, some time for relief for your system, maybe in the form of gratitude, doodling, tea, gazing at the sky, or something else. Bite-sized pieces instead of an all-at-once approach.

Advocating for New Approaches

The tide is slowly turning; the potential overwhelm that can result from exposure-based methods of meditation and therapy is being acknowledged. In an interview, David Treleaven, psychologist and researcher of trauma and mindfulness, stated that "closing your eyes and paying attention can actually exacerbate the stress that someone is experiencing. It can actually be too much.... You don't always want to go right at what's difficult" (Stang and Treleaven 2018).

I do not want to throw anyone under any buses! That is not my angle at all. I want to offer comfort to you if you are also a person who needs an easy-does-it approach. MM and EE therapies are well established, and very effective for *some people,* sometimes. But clearly *not all people.* We don't have to wonder if it is our personal shortcoming if these deep-end approaches don't work for us—it's not. And luckily, there are other ways we can recover from stress and traumas and get back to living. The pages ahead offer you an immediate start.

A Scale of 1 to 10

So when is meditating with our stress or exposure to our stress helpful? As far as administering MM or prolonged narratives, the data indicate that after mild to moderate stress is the right time. Here, a scale of 1 to 10 can be a useful guide. While a scale of 1 to 10 is a personal and subjective measure, indicating most manageable to least manageable, for simplicity's sake, 1 = mild, 5 = moderate, 10 = extreme. To add detail: 1 might be a subtle and nondisruptive experience of tension, increased awareness of discomfort, and a lack of ease; and 10 might be an unbearable reaction that might include pounding heart, tight stomach, extreme heat or extreme cold, trembling, overwhelming fear, anxiety, or panic. That puts 5 in the range of unpleasant, persistent, but mostly manageable. I've found that if a person's stress level is ranging from a 1 to a 5, meditation and talking things through can be really positive, even significantly relieving. However, if the stress level is consistently hovering between a 5 and a 10, it might be best to navigate around practices that take you into your head, often too quickly and much too deep.

Try This: Notice Your Stress Levels

Over the next week, observe your experience when your stress levels rise. Using the scale of 1 to 10— 1 being very little stress, 5 being strong but manageable stress, 10 being extreme stress—note the frequency and scale of your stress.

- When you are in (objectively) low-stress situations (low for the average person, that is), what stress levels do you *experience*?

- When you are in moderately stressful situations, what level of stress do you *experience*?

- When you are in highly stressful situations, what stress level do you *experience*?

Did you find that you are *very* stressed, even by sort of small things? (For example, you noticed your stress level was at a 7 for an objectively 3-type situation.) Or did you find that you actually got very stressed only in very stressful circumstances, but then you'd get really, *really* stressed? (For example, with an objectively 8 to 9 stress event you quickly hit a 10+ and maybe stayed there for quite a while.)

Use the form here as a model for recording in a journal or notebook.

When this situation was objectively a	Low-Stress Situation, 1 through 3	Moderate-Stress Situation, 4 through 6	High-Stress Situation, 7 through 10
Your experience of the stress level			

YOU DO YOU

Any time I hear someone trying to squeeze their round self into a square hole, I want to sit next to them and console them and help them feel— they don't have to. You don't have to force your healing. You don't have to push yourself to get better. You need patience and time, and to be round if you're round and square if you're…you get the idea. This book offers several other ways to help yourself. Several ways to be round, square, what-have-you. (And this is just the beginning; there are dozens more in the field of somatic regulation.) The MBR approach is totally the opposite of "no pain, no gain." The MBR approach is if there *is* pain, there will be *no* gain.

Why Not Stay Up in Your Head?

Why not stay up in your head? As Sapolsky (2004) points out, *thinking about* stressful things is just as alarming to our entire body-mind system as *living through* actual stressful things—meaning that mindfully witnessing our stress (meditation) or steadily describing our stress (exposure therapy) can seriously stress us out. For individuals whose body-mind systems regularly experience dysregulation, it's a simple math equation: live stress events + mental stress events = too many stress events. When there are too many instances of stress activation happening in the system, the dysregulation can become intrusive, which can be mentally and emotionally debilitating.

Van der Kolk (2014) explains that almost everyone exposed to extreme stress develops some intrusive symptoms; these are like shadows of the stress passing through your body and mind. Many studies confirm that mental and physical signals of stress, such as elevated heart rate and increased body temperature, incite intrusive memories of historic stress events to appear seemingly out of nowhere. This is an unwanted detour loop. Stress brings about unwanted stress sensations, such as heart palpitations and erratic body temperatures; then heart palpitations and erratic body temps bring about intrusive memories of stress. Around and around we go! Stress mind to stress body and then stress body to stress mind.

POTENTIAL HAZARDS TO WATCH OUT FOR

Let's take a look at three potential hazards it's important to be aware of. Don't let these go unnoticed or undersupported. These are the body-mind system's SOS—your nervous system trying to let you know that help is needed and should be called for, expeditiously.

Potential Hazard 1: Hijacking the Body-Mind

This stress loop can take a serious toll on your functioning. Stress memories can hijack your brain, leaving you stranded in stress. Van der Kolk (2014) points out that unintegrated images, sensations, thoughts, smells, and sounds of extreme stress live in a separate part of the brain from our integrated sense impressions. These stress memories seat themselves outside of the parts of the brain that help us know where we are and who we are. From within this disoriented stress brain, we don't know that a memory that is intruding in on us today is actually from the past.

Both Levine (1997, 2010) and van der Kolk emphasize that the more extreme stress you have lived through, the more your brain is trapped in the past, and the worse your brain is at noticing the truth of today. Adding insult to injury, the more extreme stress you store in your system, the more reactive your brain is to any triggers related to stress. Because memories often pop up during MM and EE therapies, and stressed brains gravitate toward stress memories, both of these methods can be like putting out the welcome mat for unintegrated fears to intrude. From the intrusion, it's easy for the stress memories to hijack us.

Break Time

Take a moment to breathe a little more deeply. Then tilt your head slowly from side to side, taking a few longer breaths with each tilt. Gentle and slow. No rush.

Next, wiggle a little, maybe your shoulders, feet, fingers, toes...breathing fully as you do. Feel your body as you move. Good for you!

Potential Hazard 2: Flooding

As I have been describing with my body-of-water metaphor, extreme stress can create a deep pool of reactivity within us. Unfortunately, the deep end of the pool can be all too easy for us to fall into and to become stuck in when stress is a regular at the poolside cabana. The term "psychological flooding" fits the deep-end metaphor very well. I think of psychological flooding as the experience of unwittingly falling into the waters of stress memory and submerging both emotionally and physically in experiences from the past. This painful submergence easily gives way to a loop of mind stress to body stress and so on.

Flooding and recoupling. It's not just the stress loop we need to be aware of where flooding is concerned. Importantly, when flooding occurs, the intrusive memories from our past can then be overlaid on whatever is happening in the present moment. When this joining takes place, neutral or even positive events and environments change for us and can seem overwhelming or hostile. Levine explains that these kinds of overlays can lead to coupling stress reactivity with what are typically nonstress events. This can then incite high levels of stress activation even in fairly neutral settings (you know—the grocery store, a business lunch, school drop-off or pick-up, a night out on the town). With stress recoupling, even activities that seem tranquil and healthy to most people can feel like danger zones to those with unprocessed extreme stress. For the extremely stressed, MM or EE therapies can be prime arenas for automatic stress reexperiencing and negative recoupling to occur.

Break Time

Again, take a few longer, fuller breaths. Then reach your arms out wide and stretch for a few breaths. Next, reach your arms up high and stretch for a few breaths. Gentle and slow. No rush. Feel your body as you move. Good for you!

Potential Hazard 3: Override

A very important addition to the commonly named three F's of stress response—flight, fight, or freeze—is social support or soothing through connection. Porges' extensive research (1996, 2014) shows that when humans feel unsafe, our *first* instincts are to try to get help and support from others. We instinctively try to engage with safe people or animals to gain safety, protection, and increased regulation *before* we attempt the three F's. If social support and safety is not available or possible to achieve, our next evolutionary response is to attempt to protect ourselves by fleeing; then we progress to self-protection through fighting. These are stages one, two, and three of our instinctual self-*preservation* and when allowed to play out, they support healthy self-regulation. Unfortunately, these stages may not be consistently supported by MM and EE therapies. For example, the absence of social support is inherent in traditional MM. The standard instructions for MM are to not talk to, be in physical contact with, or look at others while meditating. For a stressed individual needing social support, this opposes her or his evolutionarily instinctive actions for self-regulation. To follow these basic meditation instructions, the dysregulated meditator must learn to override their basic social-support instinct. Another override concerning MM can stem from the instruction to sit still, often traditionally described as being unwavering in one's posture. If a flight instinct arises for the dysregulated meditator, staying still in that meditation posture inherently requires an override of this self-preservation instinct—when an action as simple as getting up and moving freely could be enough to curtail a flashback. Levine supports the notion that even small shifts in body posture and subtle movements can help to regulate the system when a flight response arises. Without the freedom to socially connect or to physically move, sitting with and/or breathing through intrusive memories or sensations can convert meditation into a deeply troubling experience for the meditator with a history of extreme stress.

Similarly, revisiting one's stress history in EE therapies can become dysregulating. Without carefully and repeatedly interjecting somatic-regulation tools during the retelling of a stress history, the therapist can unintentionally guide the client directly into the deep end of the pool. The client can easily feel left alone to wade in the too-deep waters of their memories and forced to override their own instincts to jump out of these painful memories for a break or for shallower waters.

One longtime EE therapist who studied somatic therapy later in her career shared with me that after learning about the concepts of not getting into the stress too quickly or too deeply, she was acutely aware of how her exposure emphasis did the opposite. She explained that in her EE sessions she had often encouraged her clients to explore the difficult memories and to probe the pain that they caused. Like a runaway train, the stress memories can take the client to places she or he doesn't want to go. The pace and intensity found in EE and MM might override the client's healthy self-preservation instincts: engaging soothing social connection, fleeing from excessive stress or overwhelm, and what can be taboo but is surely sometimes very necessary, self-protecting by rejecting or fighting against that which leads to a felt experience of "this is too much."

Break Time

Enjoy a few fuller breaths and let each one out with a long, low sigh sound. Feel your belly as you sigh. Gentle and slow. No rush.

Notice the sensations in your body as you breathe and sigh. Good for you!

Potential Hazard 4: Dissociation

If none of our first three instincts—social protection, flight, or fight—is possible, as a last resort, our primitive instincts guide us to weather the threat by freezing or shutting down. This is akin to becoming like a statue and hoping no one notices you (freeze), or becoming inert and waiting for the stress-storm to pass (shutdown). Of the two—freezing or shutting down—freeze is often the initial reaction, which then progresses to shutdown if the stress event is either too long lasting or too enormous to contend with. In a freeze state, there is actually a *hyper*activation (intense internal reactivity) underneath a *hypo*reactive, statue-like exterior. In this case, the storm is not actually passing; rather, it is festering deep within the statue, only to surface again at a later time with all the same activation and intensity that created the freeze in the first place. This can easily become a cycle of activation leading to freeze, only to resurface or thaw later, leading to another freeze. According to Levine, the freeze response calls for slow, careful, and thoughtfully interjected somatic-regulation skills that help to thaw the freeze one drop at a time. The intensity of MM or EE therapies is not optimal for thawing this tender state.

Porges and Levine assert that after freeze, the next progression of self-preservation instincts is the state of collapse, whereby the system succumbs to an involuntary shutdown. In this state, there is an automatic dissociation; the MM meditator or EE client is simply gone from their body and mind for a time. With MM, this dissociation is often curtailed only by the bell ringing to indicate the mediation period's ending. I am all too familiar with hearing meditation students report that they initially felt intense struggle during the first minutes of the meditation, but "stayed with it," and felt as if they just "floated through the time." I have often heard, "I only realized time had passed when I heard the chime to end the meditation." This is a classic description of meditative dissociation. Likewise, it is all too common in EE for a person to recite a well-rehearsed stress history monologue from a state of freeze or shutdown. Clients can spend years telling their story without feeling much or any increase in self-regulation or substantial relief from intrusive symptoms.

Break Time

See something around you that you enjoy looking at. Let your eyes rest there. Next, place your hands on your belly and allow your next breath in to fill up your lungs. As you breathe out, let your lungs empty completely. Repeat several times.

When the System Normalizes Stress

If you spend too much time on any of these detours, stress can become your system's new normal. Being hijacked or flooded by stress or overriding or dissociating from self-protection instincts are all forms of reexposure to your stress pathways. Studies show that regular reexposure can erode your self-preservation capacities. Sapolsky (2004) describes a study finding that an average mouse with no history of stress can learn to defend itself against a stressor—small shocks—by learning to read the signals the scientists give off when they are about to administer the stressor. The mice with no history of stress learn how to get out of the stressor zone and instead retreat to the safe areas of their environment with no stressor—where no shocks are given. When scientists performed the same experiment with mice that had a stress history, these mice couldn't learn to get themselves to safety. They couldn't learn to read the cues that came before the small shocks—same cues for both sets of mice. Instead, they gave up and just let themselves be shocked. Anything that teaches you to sit in the activation and stress, even seemingly healthy approaches like MM and EE therapies, can contribute to this. A sad demonstration that flooding, override, and dissociation can have lasting negative consequences.

POSSIBLE WARNING NEEDED

We've seen that, although many people have been aided by MM and EE therapies, when it comes to somatic anxiety and extreme stress, we may be wise to proceed with caution. Meditation and exposure therapies might need a warning label. *Warning: Can worsen symptoms. If you experience an outbreak of stress, watch carefully for 24 to 48 hours. If symptoms persist, discontinue use and consult a somatic professional.*

It's essential here to draw a distinction between mindfulness and meditation. Mindfulness is awareness and attention; meditation is a specific application of mindful awareness, already described in preceding examples. Ellen Langer, a professor at Harvard University, has been researching mindfulness for more than thirty years. Her enormous body of work centers on mindful awareness *without* any meditation practices involved. Her studies show great results for the power of awareness, demonstrating clearly that meditation and awareness are independent skills. Awareness is central for somatic regulation; meditation is not.

ANTIDOTES

If the potential hazards above lead to an SOS call, these antidotes can be a good start to getting you headed back to smooth sailing: First, attend to sensations; next, remember to take it slow; then let your body guide you.

Antidote 1: Acknowledge What You Feel in Your Nervous System

When it comes to stressful situations and memories of them, it is not helpful to do what some of us might remember from childhood, when we didn't want to hear or see what was happening. We'd plug our ears, close our eyes, and hum *la da la da* loudly to mask out whatever is there. Our *body* very much remembers the stress, even if we try to shut tightly against the sights, sounds, and sensations. I often say to my clients (and myself), "We are going to start by slowly getting into the shallow water, and regularly take you to the edge of the water where you can catch your breath and sense your body here and now. We are not suddenly going to throw you in the deep end and see if you can stay afloat. We're dipping in a few toes, taking a rest, getting in up to your ankles, and then again reminding ourselves we have buoys at the ready." And at each of these stages, we're sensing, feeling, and knowing our bodies as they dip, and rest, and swim, and breathe.

Antidote 2: Less Is More

The "not too deep or fast" approach speaks to Levine's hugely important concept of less is more. More means going right at the problem, diving in and steeping in it, or trying to stare it down and battle it out. This causes a lot of activation in the system, often more than the stress sufferer can handle. (I mean, it was bad enough the first time, right?

Why replicate the overwhelm?) If the stress memory comes rushing in too quickly or you're in too deep, it's time for a pause. This pause will be covered much more in the skills chapters (4, 5, and 6).

Antidote 3: Lead with the Body

The body is the cornerstone of somatic stress resilience. The nervous system speaks in the language of sensation. Head-centered approaches don't communicate effectively with your nervous system; your body cannot be talked out of its reactions. Communicating with the nervous system is done from sensation to sensation, with one gentle dip in at a time. Easy does it. It's not all in your head; it's in your body too.

Try This: Brief Self-Regulating Practice

This isn't just a theory; this is our lives.

If you look over the lists of symptoms and triggers in this chapter and chapter 1 and read through situations that might be bringing you stress or tension, what do you notice your body? Right here, right now: what are you experiencing somatically?

Can you hold whatever sensations you notice within a framework of kindness? Even directing kindness toward your tension, stress, or fear? Let yourself be here for just a moment, being with your sensations with kindness.

Now, is there anywhere in your body where you feel a little bit less tense? Anywhere that is any amount more okay than another? Scan for areas where there is some slight softening, some bit of relative comfort. Those are your oases. Be with those for a moment now.

With the array of sensations in your body gently held in your awareness, can you hang out for a few breaths? Be particularly aware of what is okay, or okay *enough*.

Let this practice come to a gradual end. Now let it go completely and just be you, here and now, with no special effort of any kind.

Good for you!

CHAPTER 3

The Relief Is in Your Body

An ongoing ache in her abdomen was what Susan came to see me about. She was concerned that maybe scar tissue from a surgery she had undergone as a child was somehow flaring up. We worked slowly, with her attending to her sensations little by little. During our conversation, I was very careful to help her take many breaks from her epicenter of activation, the surgery site itself. She went back and forth between gently sensing the pain in her belly region and the painful memories associated with that, to instead focusing on a relaxing memory—she chose a really great trip she had just taken. When we talked about her trip, her body would relax, shoulders widen, face brighten, and breathing deepen, and her belly would feel ease. Then when we would revisit the surgery site and memories, the opposite would occur—jagged breath, tightening in of the shoulders, gripping in her jaw, furrowing of her brow, pain in her belly.

The contraction related to her belly and memories were made bearable by the expansion she felt when she recalled the freedom and joy of her summer travels. With each cycle of visiting the contraction and then being led out of it to the expansion, the subsequent contraction lessened and the sensations were less painful. After several rounds of this contraction-expansion cycle, Susan described that her sensations had become softer, gentler, and completely manageable. She recognized that her newly emerging sensations were a felt experience of long-ago fear. She explained that it felt as though the fear were asking for support. Susan's need for support began during the surgery itself, now more than forty years ago. But her need and vulnerability had been concealed under a tight knot we could name the "whatever it takes" knot. This knot entails one's whole mind-body system engaging and contracting to do whatever it takes to get through something—a something that is actually too much of a burden to be shouldered without system-wide flexing. Susan's flexing had been acting as armor against her completely apt pain and fear.

This one session did not resolve all of her surgery trauma; that would need more time and care. But substantial progress was made. Attending to the contractions and releases had begun to open up a new pathway for her. By moving through her body's natural cycle of tension and *recovery from tension*, the pain that had been locked in under tight constriction for so many years could lighten and give way to the previously concealed fear. Her fear could then be recognized and given the care that was needed to address and ease it.

CYCLES OF TENSION AND RELEASE

Contraction and expansion—that's how our nervous systems are designed to function. When this cycle is cut short or buried deep, as can often be the case with extreme-stress events, our recovery is also cut short and buried deep. Restoring this natural biological process returns us to our ability to complete the recovery and builds internal pathways of stress resilience.

Try This: Cycling Between Tension and Release

Take a moment to move from tension to release in your own body-mind.

1. Allow yourself some time to call to mind a *somewhat* challenging memory. Please do not go for the hardest stuff you've got. It's not wise to work with those topics on your own; for those, you'll want a copilot.

2. After you've identified a *somewhat* challenging event, turn to the other side of your memory bank and call to mind a fairly pleasing or even pretty darn nice event you've experienced recently. It doesn't have to be perfect, just generally a good-enough time.

3. With your two scenarios identified, focus in on the generally good-enough time you've selected. As you remember this time, let yourself gently feel what happens in your body. What does your chest

feel like? Your shoulders, back, or neck? How about your belly? Can you sense the rhythm of your breath? Identify some areas of your body that *feel* somewhat pleasant, or somewhere on the spectrum between pleasant and pretty okay. Let yourself take in these sensations for a few breaths. No big deal; just noticing areas of okayness in your body. Gently take in what you *feel*.

4. Now give yourself some time with the *somewhat* challenging memory. Let yourself remember how it was for you. As you call this event to mind, what happens in your body? Does your breathing change? How about the sensations in your chest, belly, back, and so on? Is it okay to stay with these sensations for a few breaths? Please, if it is too much, swing right over to the positive memory. If it is okay—not great (not expecting a fun time here), but still manageable—then hang out and attend to your sensations for a few breaths. Witness them with kindness and curiosity. Don't stay too long; less is more here.

5. Now that you have both of these body-mind destinations set up, spend a few moments swinging back and forth between these two felt experiences. Your memories might be primarily pictures in the mind, a narrative of the event, or mostly sensations. Each of us remembers things differently; one is not better than the other. However, after you're able to recognize the *current moment* sensations that are here right now, let the historical event itself be secondary. Play with moving back and forth between these scenarios with your primary attention *on the sensations that are happening here and now*. See if you recognize the movement from tightness to a more relaxed bodily experience. Slowly swinging from side to side like a Mobius loop, infinitely connected—pulling in, extending out, tightening, loosening, contracting, releasing.

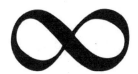

BODY CONTRACTIONS

As I've been saying, our response to extreme stress takes place primarily in our bodies—with a dusting of mental worry and rumination on top. This snow-capped mountain of reactivity, which we will break down further in the following sections, has extreme constriction at its core. Extreme constriction means holding in, clamping down, and shutting tight—the solid rock at the core of this mountain of stress is as hard as granite during periods like these.

Tension and contraction are how we humans involuntarily respond to stress. It happens from head to toe. Our vision sharpens and we zero in on the problem—a.k.a. tunnel vision. Our salivary glands constrict, creating dry mouth. Our muscles squeeze, leading to a reflexive clench in the jaw, knotting in the belly, or gripping in of the shoulders, thighs, and butt. There can be clamping in the legs and cramping in the feet, just to name some of the automatic contractions that occur under stress.

Try This: How Does Your System Contract?

Pause for a moment to see if you recognize constriction in your own response to stress. Do you notice that your mouth regularly goes dry when you're face to face with difficulty? Do you find yourself stuck in tunnel vision, missing what else might be going on? How about bowel tension, leading to diarrhea, constipation, or a cycle of both? Do you suffer from symptoms like ongoing neck, back, or leg pain due to muscle tightness? Do you grind your teeth? Are stress headaches common for you?

What other signs of system-wide contraction are you familiar with? Making a note of these can help you to recognize when and where your body might be going into stress autopilot. Recognizing when stress reactions are taking place will be a key step to guiding yourself back out of the reaction and off of the stress autobahn.

Overwhelming Helplessness

There is one state of body-mind that, if unresolved, often creates lasting stress imprints. When imprinting takes place, the stress reaction becomes inscribed into your muscles, nerves, gut, heart, and brain. That state is *overwhelm.*

When I consulted a thesaurus for synonyms for overwhelm to help me better flesh out this concept, I found *devastated, overpowered,* and *helpless.* Yup, that's what we're talking about here.

Overwhelm plays a huge role in how stress, especially extreme stress, affects us. Overwhelm comes in all shapes and sizes.

It overtook Rachel when her husband suddenly announced that he wanted a divorce and shockingly revealed his infidelity during their twenty-year marriage.

Melinda's overwhelm overtook her while she was standing in front of several hundred esteemed colleagues and students at a prestigious university. While lecturing in her area of expertise, she was feeling plagued by insecurities, self-criticism, and the terror that they would all see right through her act of composure—she then went completely blank and had to end midway through the lecture.

Eric was overcome by helplessness while rushing his son to the emergency room. He had witnessed the accident from only a few feet away, yet too far away to stop it from happening.

For Beth, overwhelm came as anger and bewilderment at seeing her daughter somehow become the target of what could be called childhood social experimentation but left her little one teased, rejected, and alone.

If during your stress events you've felt not only the pressure and constriction that are inherent in extreme stress, but were also left feeling helpless, devastated, or overpowered, you would have been in a state of overwhelm. It is essential that any of us who enter this state recover from it. If we do not, there will be lasting stress imprints. Just as our body-mind system is designed to go from contraction to expansion, as we've discussed, it is also designed to go through the natural process of *moving through* feeling overpowered to feeling powerful again. If recovery does not take place, this state of overwhelm can become chronic, and a chronic state becomes a *trait.* A state is like the new seed, and the trait is like the years-old vine, weaving around everything in your garden.

As a trait, overwhelm becomes part of the way you function in the world. And this trait can be an invasive vine that begins to strangle all your other cultivated plants. We can interrupt this invasion if we can restore the natural cycles—contraction and expansion, overpowered and powerful, stress and resilience—within the body-mind system. With this return to natural biology, we keep a state of overwhelm as it was meant to be—temporary. Temporary overwhelm, while difficult to bear, does not embed. It will not become part of how you exist in the world. Restoring the cycle of activation and deactivation in your body-mind establishes what was missing from your stress events of years gone by—a beginning, middle, and end.

Imprints

When persistent felt experiences of not being able to deal with what you are facing embed deeply in your nervous system, you are experiencing stress imprinting. Much as a glacier can carve deep and enduring ruts through towering mountains as the mass of ice persistently bears down on the range, stress imprints can carve paths into your nervous system. What was meant to be only a situationally relevant state of overwhelm can become an unyielding trait of overwhelm that overlays on all kinds of situations—whether it's relevant or necessary or not. When stress imprints repeatedly dictate your reactions, lightning-speed tremors of contraction and fear become your new normal. This becomes embodied stress, anxiety, and overwhelm. In this mode, it feels like whatever is going on is too much—waaayyy too much. It's not that your *brain* actually thinks there is something terribly wrong as you shop the aisles in the supermarket, wait in traffic, attend meetings, go out on a first date—it's your *body* that has taken over and taken you into a whole-body reaction that stems from deep stress imprinting.

Imprints and Baseline

During each repeated episode of embodied stress, anxiety, and overwhelm, the stress becomes more and more normal to your body. If very high levels of stress reactivity become the norm, this can reset your baseline, and your stress scale, ranging from 1 to 10, can get way out of whack. When your baseline is reset, instead of functioning at a 2 or 3 for average daily events, your body might perform at a 7 or 8 stress level just to open the mail. This creates a destination of stress so imprinted that it can be hard *not to* hop on that superhighway and head to Stressville whenever things start to *feel* amped up.

If your baseline isn't very base, stress is how you do your day. The MBR protocol that I developed for my research study reset the participant's baselines; this is the protocol found in this book. By incorporating the settling and soothing methods in the coming chapters into your daily routines, your body can create a very new normal, one that leaves you feeling at ease, trusting, and comfortable in your own skin. With stress resilience, instead of the solid ice of the stress glaciers, we will facilitate melting, and then softening of the whole stress mountain. And instead of feelings of helplessness that painfully linger, they'll have a beginning, middle, and end.

For those who have spent long periods feeling helpless and unable to cope, our stress imprints don't just show up during major stress events; they have haunted us in all kinds of other moderate or even mild stress situations—precisely because they don't seem to have an end, they just travel with us from life event to life event. As we restore our body's evolutionary disposition to respond to stress—*and then recover from it*—we will come out from under the heavy weights of chronic tension and overwhelm. We will return to the resilience that evolution means for us to have.

FEELING RESILIENCE

Feeling your resilience and recovery is essential to resetting your baseline and directing yourself away from Stressville. Without physically knowing your recovery from stress, your body-mind system can miss it—and often does. Unfortunately, with extreme stress, the felt experience of returning to regulation is, well, easy to miss. The stress can be so loud, it can be hard to hear the quieter tones of resilience. To the body-mind, if we miss the *experience* of stress recovery, it can be as if the recovery never happened.

If your system doesn't register that you've transitioned from threat to safety, evolution causes your primitive brain to assume you're still under threat. It's as if you are still standing behind the bushes on lookout duty, waiting and waiting for the predator to arrive, so you can *finally* defend yourself and move on. If you don't have a visceral feeling of successful defense or escape, followed by moving on, you don't move on.

As Levine and Sapolsky have pointed out, we can take a lesson from the evolutionary smarts of those kings and queens of the jungle, the lions. Levine and Sapolsky were both brilliant in their observations of animals' successful stress recovery as a model for our own. Picture this example of successful defense and escape, followed by full-bodied recovery and rest. A beautiful lioness has just successfully chased away a pack of hyenas. After she has secured her safety and assessed that she is indeed out of danger, she finds a nice shady spot under some trees. Then she circles in the grass until it is tamped down just so. She licks her paws a few times and crosses them in front of her, creating a pillow for her head. Finally, she leisurely lets out a big wide yawn, lays her weary head on her paws, and *rests*.

As she lies there, her breathing and body temperature will return to normal. Her heart rate will become steady again. Her muscles will relax. Eyes, ears, and throat will relax. Her internal organs will unclench and resume their jobs again. She has skillfully followed a full cycle from contraction to release, from stress to recovery, from temporary overwhelm (or at least a high state of "whelm") to again feeling powerful.

We would be wise to settle into a nice cozy spot and catch our breath after we overcome our hurdles. Our nervous systems would thank us mightily.

Try This Later: Feel Your Resilience

The next time you encounter a *moderate* stress event, try bringing your awareness to what's *okay* in your body. Do this a little during the event, and *a lot* after it's all over. Initially, the stress event might automatically trigger responses like rapid breathing, increased body temperature, muscle tension, dry mouth, and cloudy thinking.

- During the event, notice if there are any areas of your body that are just a little less tense than the primary areas of tension; even just a bit of ease can help. Maybe the muscles in your hands are less tense than another part of your body. Perhaps you can feel that your legs are less hot than your chest or face.

- After the event has passed, you can really take in the process of your body's calming down and returning to a regulated state. See if you can feel your breathing returning to a deeper, more rhythmic cycle. Notice the sensations of tension releasing from your muscles, gut, or mind. Observe your heart rate slowing and body temperature returning to a more comfortable degree. I suggest to my clients: get into this experience like you would get into a hot tub on a cool brisk night—ease your way in, then really soak in it for a few moments. Enjoy your recovery; your amazing body-mind system deserves it.

Listening for the Quiet of Recovery

A person who has been in a nearly fatal car accident and subsequently lives with persistent anxiety is trapped in the "noise" of the incident—the persistent experience of hyper- or hypoactivation can feel like the static noise displayed on a TV screen with no signal occurring constantly beneath your skin. One client spent a few years with ongoing trembling after her own brush with trauma. While her muscular tension, elevated heart rate, and digestive shutdown may lessen just enough to make her appear functional, if her body-mind system doesn't *experience* the bodily tension decreasing, heart slowing, gut returning to being open for business, and finally a settled stillness within the whole mind-body system, it can be as if this de-escalation never took place.

If her body-mind system is not updated and the end of the overwhelming event not registered, even a slight stressor can trigger all the reactivity that sprang forth during the car accident to resurface and repeat all over again. To this system, it feels as if the accident is still happening. It's as if the noise of fear is persisting without any quiet for recovery. Without having carried out her entire resilience cycle through *feeling its completion,* within her primitive brain, the threat is not gone.

Chronic Noise of Stress

Sometimes the noise of our stress just keeps playing, seeming to never end, drowning out the quiet return to okayness. With chronic or too-often-repeated stressors, where there isn't a clear before, during, and after, it can be even more important to notice *and sense* any "silence between the notes" that might occur.

Persistent noise of stress can come from both large and small strings of events. The event is not the signal of dysregulation. How your body-mind reacts to it—and whether it recovers from it—is the key to regulation or lack thereof. For a student I assisted in the Somatic Experiencing training, it went something like this. Although she was a professional in her early fifties, like many students, she was in debt and living modestly. As luck would have it, her car broke down the day before she was to drive to the training. "I can deal with this," she thought, and rented a car for the week. While driving the rental car, she noticed it wasn't running very well. Before long she found herself waiting by the side of the road for a replacement rental. "I've got this," she thought, and pressed on.

When she finally arrived at her Airbnb rental, the place was a mess and felt unsafe to her. "I can't stay here for my training week," she lamented to herself. She trudged on and rented a hotel room. Her confidence that things were going to be okay was eroding. This had become a string of surprising, disappointing, and difficult hurdles for her to cross. She entered the training raw and emotional, afraid and edgy (completely understandable!). It wasn't until three days into the training that she realized she had been completely stuck in hyperactivation. She only realized how high and persistent her activation had been after a moment of *slightly* less activation.

As she sat across from me, she was experiencing a slight downshift in her system and some relief that, in that moment, felt long overdue. Luckily she caught the experience of her morsel of relief, deeply noticed it, and took it in. Until that moment, her recovery hadn't yet happened. Too many stressors had piled up in a row, like being in the jungle and seeing one tiger after another pursuing you. She hadn't been able to feel any middle or end to her reactivity, only beginning after beginning. Now, days into her stress reaction, some recovery finally was taking place; an end was occurring within her. With tears running down her cheeks, she said, "I'm sure I would have remained stuck in this sky-high activation were it not for being here at this somatic training. I feel so lucky that this was where I was driving to when it all began."

Before *feeling* some of the pressure release, like air being let out of a balloon, she had been ready to pop. Among other things, she had been struggling to keep her primitive or stress brain from overtaking her modern or complex-thinking brain. (The modern brain is so called because it evolved some 200,000 years ago, whereas the primitive brain evolved approximately 500,000 years ago.) Her complex-thinking brain knew she was at a training, staying in a nice-enough hotel, and driving a working-enough car. But her primitive brain was still hiding in the bushes, looking for where the next tiger would be coming from.

The Importance of Moving On

Sapolsky points out the master plan evolution made for us: to be able to respond with enormous strength, endurance, and focus to overcome *short-lived* stressors. We were wired for fleeting reactivity, like running from predators or protecting our harvest from storms and then to be done with it. Maybe even to rest—or like the lioness, to have a casual yawn, at the very least. We need time to shift from that narrow survival focus to a broader, more relaxed, more nuanced view and sense of things.

This is evolution's gift of a stage we could call "moving on." Moving on from supercharged stress levels. Moving on from system-wide contraction. Moving on from survival, so we don't live as if the house were constantly on fire. When we are running on all cylinders and jump in headfirst but circumnavigate the "cool your jets" part of the plan, we get ourselves into a lot of trouble—the likes of the illness and dysregulation described in chapter 1. We're not wired for decades-long stressors. We bring "let's do this" instincts to "slow your roll" situations. And when we are all action, we miss the all-important *silence* between the notes that makes the music beautiful—as the French composer Debussy is said to have observed, "Music is the space between the notes." A composition without any space between the notes is just noise.

PHYSICAL PROBLEM, PHYSICAL SOLUTION

Just as we cannot mentally demand that our physical reactions begin—we can't successfully order: "Heart, begin to race; mouth, go dry"—we also cannot mentally demand that they end. And until that solid ice of stress melts or at least significantly softens, our persistent stress reactions will continue to be all-too-frequent guests—the kind that come too often and stay too long, leave their dirty laundry on the floor and crumbs on the counter near the toaster (grrrr!), and of course are too noisy.

Instead of trying to mentally change a physical issue, let us enter into the resolution of these physical symptoms through the doorway in which they began: the body. Start in the body, and stop in the body. After all, why would we try to get to the ocean by walking toward the desert? We're trying to walk toward the ocean of our own bodies, and we each get there through our own *interoception*.

INCREDIBLE INTEROCEPTION

Intero-what? Interoception—a multisyllabic scientific word meaning feeling what's happening in your body—is incredible. Having a felt sense of your internal experience turns out to be a wonder tool for increasing regulation and returning to functional activation and deactivation—physical problem, physical solution. However, for the purposes of self-regulation, it won't work to just offhandedly notice whatever you happen to be feeling in your body. Many if not most of us don't particularly notice much of anything concerning our bodily sensations until there is an ache of some kind or something seems to be going wrong inside. In service of regulation, we turn this tendency around. Instead of our usual "I never really felt my knees until they began to hurt," we learn *regulating* interoception, distinctly noticing what *doesn't* hurt. Regulating interoception could be described simply as sensing okayness in your body. Might sound simple, but to the autonomic nervous system, it's amazing.

When you feel your body from the inside, you can remind the body-mind system about aspects of now—which normally you would have missed—that are good, or at least good enough. Whether you are noticing a part of your gut that is neutral or even comfortable, attending to sensations in your legs and arms that are somewhere between okay and pleasant, or feeling the sensations on your skin that are even somewhat pleasing, this all stands to remind your system that parts of you are fairly okay—particularly when things in that moment *are* fairly okay.

In addition to using regulating interoception when life is pretty much just humming along—which is very beneficial to your nervous system and should not be underestimated—we will also learn to use regulating interoception when things are not very okay—or not *feeling* very okay, that is. (One of the dirty tricks dysregulation plays on us is that lots of things and places can feel like danger zones, even when they really aren't.) When we are dysregulated and activated—whether from real or imagined causes—we automatically seek to find a problem. And evolution has us scanning for danger, real or imagined, whenever we feel things could (possibly, maybe...) be heading south. Part of that automatic scanning is unconscious *internal scanning* for tension, fear, stress, and other signs of activation.

To regulate ourselves when this unconscious *internal* negative bias takes hold, we can consciously *scan for okayness* in moments of distress. Using regulating interoception in times like these isn't Pollyanna-ish; it's actually seeing a fuller picture. I call it the "and also." When we are under extreme stress, there is sure to be discomfort and tension, but there is *also* usually some comfort—or at least some neutral sensations—occurring too. Even just noticing small areas of okayness can help a great deal with your well-being—a little ease in your elbow or some contentment in your foot can be meaningful messages of regulation to your body-mind.

We're not pretending that the stress isn't there. We're not ignoring it or denying it—not at all. We're just not zeroing in *only* on *it*. When we acknowledge what is not okay *and* recognize what is okay, this is the "and also" practice. Tunnel vision that sees only danger and discomfort sends you headlong into *more* stress, and, as Lao Tzu is said to have said, "If you do not change direction, you may end up where you're heading."

This change in direction redirects your system away from a much too frequent residence in Stressville. Research shows that by using this simple action, paired with the other tools in the upcoming chapters—and with patience and persistence—you will likely find your system routed away from Stressville. MBR participants describe traveling toward new destinations like this: "I can cope much more often"; "I'm not as overtaken by my stress as I used to be"; "I'm not finding myself as scared/achy/spaced out/sweaty/nauseous/angry/anxious (hyper- or hypo-activated) as I was before."

Try This: Sensing What's Okay

Here and now, take a few full breaths and let yourself get as comfortable as possible. Sitting, standing, or lying down, can you rest into your posture in a way that feels best for you? Become aware of your body as a whole, sensing yourself here in this moment. Take your time; there is no rush. Now scan your body to see if there are any areas that feel fairly okay, or even just neutral. Notice what those areas are like. Attend to the sensations there. Let those sensations land. What are they like? How do they feel now?

Continue noticing any areas of your body that feel okay and now add this awareness. How has paying attention to your okay sensations affected other areas of your body? Noticing if there are other areas of your body that are also somewhat okay or neutral. Areas that are *becoming* okay as you explore pleasant sensations. No need to look for or try to produce anything in particular. Just noticing. Sometimes awareness of okayness begets more okayness. Breathe with what you sense here for a few moments. Take as much or a little time as you would like to. Whenever you're ready, conclude this exercise.

YOUR BRAIN AND SENSATION

Sensation is the language of the nervous system. Sensations link our nervous system's instinctual back brain to our complex-thinking front brain—our primitive brain to our modern brain. Recent data in neuroscience tell us that the middle area of our frontal brain has a predisposition toward two very different tasks when "at rest." At rest means when you are not asking your brain to think about or perform specific mental activities. Science suggests when the middle brain is not on a specific assignment, it will likely devote itself to one of the following: internal dialogue *or* sensation awareness.

One option for your middle front brain is self-referential thinking. But not just any self-referential thinking; Gusnard et al. (2001) show it is likely to be a self-evaluative, even inner-critic type thinking. Your middle front brain is busy when you are "at rest." It is internally talking to you. Your resting brain is highly adept at practicing things you might say to others in the future, recounting events that had an intense effect on you from the past, and churning over countless shoulda, woulda, couldas.

Gusnard and colleagues called it an inner rehearsal. But I probably didn't need to tell you that. Spend a few minutes with your brain alone "at rest" and you are likely to be pulled into a long conversation (with yourself) about what your brain thinks about you, and what you *did* say to so-and-so, what you *should* have said to so-and-so, and oh yeah, that time you ran in to so-and-so and such-and-such happened…do I need to go on?

Luckily, your middle front brain also has a quite different skill set. It seems to also be responsible for a wide range of sensory information— receiving and processing your felt experience both from inside and outside your body. This part of your brain knows when your gut is relaxed and comfortable, or conversely, tied in knots. It also tracks when your back is in a particularly uncomfortable position while seated on that chair, or has found an easeful posture instead. It's constantly taking in cues from the sensations in your chest, the temperature on your skin, or the dryness in your mouth. Then this area of your middle brain does something profound from a self-regulation standpoint. It communicates all this sensory information to your primitive brain, sending little telegrams of okayness or not-okayness.

Circle back to incredible interoception, and you have this: sensing your okay body *while at rest* will dispatch something like a telegram to your primitive brain that all is well and it can stay in a resting state. Expand this: sensing your okay body *during and after stress* events will also send valuable telegrams to your primitive brain. In opposition to regulating interoception, we've got talking to yourself mentally, but this is not just any inner commentary. Your brain, while supposedly at rest, can go on and on about what you said wrong or should have said right (ugh!). Judging will send quite a different telegram to your primitive brain. Which kinds of messages would you like to dispatch more often:

messages of inner niggling from internal critics, or messages of areas of your body where you can rest and catch your breath?

Interoception is your brain's friend. With soothing awareness, we create foundational building blocks. First, these building blocks are made up of moments of *calming the brain before* any stress event has even occurred. Then we progress to using *sensation awareness after* stress events are over: feeling the recovery process, calming our brain, and easing our nervous system back down from its activated state. And to *interrupting stress during stress events* with sensing okayness—sometimes it's only the toes or elbows that feel okay, but we'll take it. As we do this, we slow down the writing and sending of alarming telegrams to our survival brain. Sensation awareness before, after, and even during stress events is a key to increasing resilience and well-being.

I remember two easily comparable stress events that took place during different stages of my own hard-earned resilience pathway overhaul. The first happened right in the midst of my most dysregulated period, the second at the beginning of my resilience stage. What follows is an example of a moderate stressor—a great training ground for a wide range of stress reactions. Because once you've experienced persistent extreme stress, even *moderate stressors* can trigger an *extreme stress reaction;* we're working with the same biology, whether a stress event is small, medium, or large, so we begin with the less-intense ones so as not to overwhelm ourselves.

I think you'll see, as I did, markedly different stress-recovery capacities in these different stages of my own journey of dysregulation and resilience. In both of these scenarios, I was pulled over by a police officer (I'm not a terrible driver, truly —and neither resulted in a ticket, really!). One day, I was driving home when I came to a "California stop" on my dead-end road, where no other cars were present—or so I thought. Up the block, about halfway, there was *one* other car on the otherwise empty street (I know, I know, I'm trying to justify myself). It was a police car. I'm sure he could see my horror from down the road. He looked concerned even as he pulled me over. Completely uncontrollably, I went into full force stress reactivity. I was hyperventilating, sweating, and totally red from what felt like head to toe. I could hardly get my license out of my wallet, my hands were trembling so much. Of course, I didn't want a ticket, but this reaction was *far* beyond that fear. This felt like life or death. This was what stress did to me, in me, and all over me, back in those days. He gave me a warning and sent me on my way—probably hoping I'd get out of there and safely home before I spontaneously combusted right in front of him!

Luckily, for the sake of scientific study, I was fortunate enough to be pulled over again a few years later, and several numbers lower on my baseline stress level scale. This time I was pulled over, effectively for tuning my radio, but I was being queried about looking at my cell phone (again, I'm innocent). Happily (on so many levels) I had a very different experience. This second time I had developed some stress resilience. I pulled over, began to feel my heart beat fast, and immediately invited my attention to my feet on the floor of my car and my butt on the seat. I felt my breath catch, and I explored where I felt any softening in my ribs so as to allow a fuller, easier breath to take place. I quickly checked my reflection in the rear view mirror (this was for science, people), and gave myself a little moment of celebration that I wasn't lit up like the Fourth of July. I talked to the officer, was released, and then sat in my car for a few moments and basked in all my glory. I was so happy that I hadn't gone from a stress level of 2 straight to a 10 when I saw the flashing blue and red lights that I got out of my car and did a little happy walk along the sidewalk for a few moments. It just felt so good to not be totally freaked out, as I had been a few years earlier in the same situation. I wanted my whole body-mind to remember every moment of it. I sat in that experience as if it were the nicest of hot tubs on a gorgeous winter night under the moon and stars. It was the tools you're finding in this book, and the assistance of a few really amazing Somatic Experiencing therapists, that helped me construct the resilience pathways I now have.

Regulating interoception is used throughout the MBR protocol. We circle back to regulating interoception again and again within each skills practice, and it is described as a stand-alone tool in chapter 4. Regulating interoception is part of how you can increase okayness during neutral events, reduce excessive stress reactivity within somewhat charged events, and facilitate an embodied somatic recovery after a high-stress event. Incredible interoception has a part in each step of your somatic stress recovery.

THE MBR PROTOCOL

As I developed the protocol for an MBR research study to investigate four primary tools for increasing self-regulation and decreasing anxiety and stress, sensation awareness was the glue that connected all the tools together. I chose each of these tools because they are all backed by hard science and have been tested using rigorous methods. In brief, MBR participants learned the same tools and science you have in your hands with this book. The original pilot study was conducted via a six-week course I taught with weekly hour and a half long classes. The news was good: the tools worked! The participants in my small but mighty research study all found relief from their stresses using the protocol you'll study in chapters 4 through 7. They learned to send regulating telegrams to their stress brain. These tools helped them strengthen their interoceptive abilities, calm their primitive brain, and rescue their system from the brink.

Next, I taught the protocol to several weekend retreat groups who met for three days of classes. At the same time, I was teaching these skills individually to the clients in my private practice. Each group has been able to develop these resilience tools that you are now learning.

I chose these tools because they are backed up by hard science. Each tool has been found to be successful in numerous studies conducted by scientists all over the world with participants from all walks of life.

In the original study, my study participants unanimously reported a decrease in their stress and anxiety levels. When asked to describe their before-and-after experiences, these were two of the responses.

"Before the six-week study, my stress felt static and unchanging, like a snag on a nail, always there and bothersome. Now at the end of the study, I've been able to use techniques to stop anxiety attacks. This is amazing; these tools are really effective."

"Before the study, I was really hard on myself; I felt brittle and had a lot of rumination and self-judgment. Now I have much more awareness of my physical state. I have less reactivity and less rumination."

I also chose to measure before-and-after levels of cortisol, a commonly studied stress hormone. When stress occurs in healthy and regulated populations, studies show that the body secretes cortisol, elevating levels temporarily, but then cortisol returns to normal after the stress has passed. In cases where stress occurs too often or is too unmanageable, cortisol levels do not return to normal. Even well after the stress has passed, cortisol levels remain chronically elevated, and the individuals become likely sufferers of dysregulation.

If cortisol levels were changed by the MBR course, it would show that not only did thoughts and feelings change as a result of MBR, but *physiology* could be changed by the tools. The group showed remarkable results. Every participant's cortisol levels dropped, meaning *all* their physiological stress levels went down. The average cortisol drop for my research group was 41 percent. As is common in small research studies, these results were used to generate estimates of what we might see in larger groups. A well-respected and widely used tool for data analysis—Cohen's d—showed that in a group of 100 volunteers who learned the MBR tools, 96 would have reliable cortisol reduction. For research, those are excellent results!

I'll briefly mention the tools here—a little sneak peek before you investigate more deeply in each skills chapter. However, the ultimate investigation is inside yourself.

Tool #1: Rhythmical Breathing

Breathing your nervous system back into balance will be covered in chapter 4. An MBR participant reported, "The breathing really works for me; it resets my psyche and brings me back to a *not* freaked out state." Because stress easily interrupts our natural breathing rhythm, this chapter provides a few options for rhythmical breathing; each can be custom fitted to your unique needs.

Tool #2: Seeing and Sensing

Chapter 5 will teach you how to stay in, or return to, the here and now—which is not as straightforward as it sounds. When you are confronted with a *real-life stress event,* and when your real life is reminding you of a *previous stress event,* dysregulation can easily take you far, far away from present-day reality. One study participant said, "When I practiced seeing outside in nature, I became *really* present. It has helped me several times, and each time I feel proud of myself for coming back to now."

Tool #3: Imagery for Self-Regulation

Chapter 6 will guide you to use internal images to create ease instead of stress, the third primary tool. Working with pictures in the mind, which just pop up for many of us when remembering stress events, you'll learn how to facilitate deep relief for your mind-body system. One research study participant described it this way: "I saw myself replay flashes of negative images and *felt* the reactivity from them playing." After working with these images using the tools in chapter 6, she said, "After two *really* weird days I was actually able to relax."

Tool #4: Movement

Chapter 7 will teach simple movement to calm your nervous system through your internal braking system—the vagus nerve. These easy stretches can significantly help restore ease to your body-mind system and curtail the tightness and statue-like stillness that can often accompany stress reactivity. During the six-week study, one participant shared, "At first I was feeling stuck, total inertia." By week six, she shared delightedly, "This time I felt my *whole* back release. That *doesn't* often happen for me."

Try This: Breathing, Sensing, Seeing Okayness

- Take a moment now to easily breathe. Next, tip your head from side to side. Allow your neck to gently stretch on each side and let a few longer slower breaths move in and out.

- Close your eyes and feel where in the body you are at ease, or comfortable—even just somewhat. Sense whatever level of comfort you have. Breathe with what you notice.

- Next, bring your head back up to center. Then open your eyes and slowly look right until your head is facing the right side of the room (or space where you are). Do the same to the left.

- While you do this, let your eyes see what is around you. Notice if there is anything lovely around you, or anything your eyes enjoy seeing. Rest your gaze there for a moment. Notice your body sensations.

- When you feel ready, end this exercise.

You've read about the involuntary processes of tension, overwhelm, and imprinting. You've covered the essential elements of this journey of feeling your resilience, attending to the quiet experiences of your recovery, and intentionally sensing your mind-body system as it moves out of reactivity. With a foundation of interoceptive awareness, we now transition to the most important part of this tool kit, the *experience* of your *visceral relief*—relief from the far-too-heavy burdens of stress, anxiety, and overwhelm.

For me, it was deeply helpful to learn about the process of somatic recovery, and I've seen it be helpful for some of the people who come to me for individual sessions, classes, and retreats. Yet in all cases, the most important part of your recovery from stress, anxiety, and overwhelm is your *felt experience* of your relief. In the upcoming skills chapter, you'll still find some of the background thinking and science behind each tool. However, I encourage you to devote most of your time to *experiencing* each tool, because it is not all in your head but in your body too; it is from *within* your own mind-body system that you can guide yourself back to well-being.

CHAPTER 4

Breathing Your Way out of Stress

All right, fellow stress sufferer; now we try out some tools. The first three chapters were a lot of looking at how our mind-body works and how stress can lead to serious trouble both above and below the neck. This chapter and the three that follow take you into your body to create access to escape routes when stress is trailing you too closely (damn tailgater that it can be). These chapters will also help you build internal pathways of relief—strong resilience pathways, *embodied recovery* routes that are at the ready when you've just had it with all the pressure buildup.

This is an *in the body* job here; we can't simply think our way through this. And yet, funnily enough, for many people, knowing the basis of these tools really helps how the tools *feel* for them and, most importantly, how they *work* for them. Here it is again: the need for balance between body and mind.

I'll guide you through embodied practices at the start of each skill chapter, midway, and at the end, to support your felt understanding of these tools. I'll sandwich these practices with some biology, evolution, and scientific evidence to serve your mental understanding and, I hope, circle down to your body to aid your overall connection to the tools. The intention is to travel into your body, up to your head, back to your body and around again—unifying your mind-body system, attending to both your sensations and thoughts, and, ultimately, becoming whole again.

Try This: Slow and Low Breathing

Take a moment right now for a few slow and low breaths.

1. Get as comfortable as possible.

2. Place your hand on your belly gently and see if your can help your belly to relax.

3. Invite your next breath to be nice and slow, and very comfortable; no strain.

4. Let your breath fill up your chest and ribcage. Let your belly puff out while this breath comes in. Imagine filling up your belly like inflating a balloon.

5. Let your exhale be long and complete, gently drawing the belly in as you exhale, releasing and letting all that breath empty out, deflating the imaginary balloon.

6. Keep softening your belly as you breathe in, easily inflating and deflating the lungs with each breath cycle. Repeat this a few times. Easy does it. No strain. Just relaxed slow and low breaths.

7. After a few breath cycles, notice how you feel. If there is any stress or strain, do less on the next round. This should be easy and light. This is just allowing your body to fully breathe.

Good for you! Enjoy!

Now take a moment to feel how those breaths impacted your body-mind system. Do you feel any ease as a result of that breathing break? I invite you to keep playing around with your breathing rhythm, maybe over the course of a day or a few days. Explore your breathing rhythm with an intention to find an ally in your breath, a partner in stress recovery and well-being.

The breath can be a wonderful doorway into your body's reactions to threat or safety, aloneness or connection, stress or resilience. By walking through this doorway, we not only can *witness* the breath but have *agency* and take action to gently guide our breath out of hyper- or hypoactivation and toward more optimal states of being. This tool and the others in this book give you opportunities to *respond* to your body-mind's need for assistance with coming back to center, back to safety, and back to ease of well-being. It's not enough to just know we are tipping away from center and falling toward distress, fear, or even panic; we need simple, direct solutions in these moments of disequilibrium. Your breath is one such direct solution.

We're always breathing. It can be as simple as taking a breath in and letting a breath out. Unfortunately, it's not always so seamless. And how your breathing occurs has a tremendous effect on how your whole body-mind functions.

Just as the deep-sea diver carries a tank of oxygen, we have to carry the kernel of our individual growth with us into the world. Whatever we achieve inwardly will change outer reality.

—Anaïs Nin, inspired by Otto Rank

WHAT TAKES YOUR BREATH AWAY

For many of us, stress takes our breath away. And our breath being taken away in this context brings on more stress. This is not the kind of being swept off your feet you're likely to enjoy. What happens to *your* breathing when things are going awry? Do you hold your breath? Pant? Wheeze? Sometimes labored breathing can be like a clue in a mystery movie. A sign that you need your own help, the breath is like a warning bell signaling you're tipping toward trouble—the trouble being body-mind stress reactivity.

Gasping for air. That's what stood out most from Sonya's initial symptoms of hyperactivation. Her body would involuntarily hyperventilate each time she would describe or even think too deeply about the stresses in her life. She would gasp, and explain that her throat felt tight, then say between gulps of air, "I just…can't catch…my breath." This happened often throughout our initial sessions. It was so uncomfortable for her. I wanted so badly to help.

To Sonya's delight—and mine—this strained breathing did not persist for her. Over time, as her body regulated, her stresses began to feel less looming. As her reactivity changed, her breathing changed too—for the better. Many of her circumstances were still the same, but with increased stress resilience her body didn't fly into full reactivity with each trigger. As I've said in previous chapters, our bodies become "too good" at stress reactivity, and high-powered reactivity becomes our system's go-to for both big *and* small upsets. Breathing was not the whole enchilada for Sonya, but it was an important piece of the puzzle. I'm guessing breathing won't be the whole enchilada for you either, but it's a very helpful dish to add to the meal.

Sonya first learned to breathe more fully when she *wasn't* stressed; she then was able help her body continue breathing even when stresses *were* occurring. We're going to cover these two types of breathing in the chapter. Little by little, as stress resilience grew within Sonya—through the slow and low breathing you'll be reading about in a few pages—it became easier for Sonya to recall stressful memories or be in stressful circumstances while still being able to breathe. She then learned to use her breath to help her through challenging events as they were happening—which you'll read about in the rescue breathing section up ahead. As they helped Sonya, the skills in this chapter can help you recover your ability to nourish your system with plenty of oxygen through full, relaxed respirations.

While Sonya's body had a very pronounced somatic reaction to stress that involved constriction around her lungs and diaphragm, many of us can feel how our own breathing is compromised when we are activated by stress. If stress is ongoing or extreme, it can feel as if we haven't had a full and relaxed breath in a very long time. After learning the breathing tools in this chapter, one MBR participant said, "This new way that I'm breathing feels like the first truly deep breaths I've taken in years."

WHEN WE'RE NOT BREATHING ENOUGH

When we can't seem to get enough air, it alarms our system. Our blood oxygen levels become skewed by under- or over-breathing, and this turns on our stress physiology, directly exacerbating our stress experience. When blood oxygen levels are thrown off, we can have symptoms like cold hands and feet, light-headedness, dizziness, even fainting, and, of course, anxiousness.

Why does our stress body keep us from full yet relaxed breaths? The stress-induced systemic contraction I explained in chapter 3 is a big part of it. The body-wide constriction that occurs during a stress response tightens the muscles throughout the torso, squeezing the lungs. Under this strain, the diaphragm is quickly affected, causing our breathing to be almost instantaneously altered by stress. This entire circus is sending thousands of signals from our lung region to our brain about whether we are okay or not okay and whether it is time to call in the troops for auxiliary support. These troops would be either the sympathetic or the parasympathetic troops, two distinct branches of your nervous system. To explain the importance of these troops, we'll need to take a trip to your vagus.

A TRIP TO YOUR VAGUS

While I've been talking a lot about fight or flight, which is part of a *sympathetic response* to stress, there is another side to this coin: the parasympathetic response. The *parasympathetic response* is related to your recovery from stress, sometimes referred to as a return to resting and digesting. The parasympathetic response is also described as tending and befriending, which I'll talk about more in chapter 8. Resting and digesting as well as tending and befriending both involve your vagus.

Your vagus nerve (or tenth cranial nerve, if counting nerves is your thing) runs from your brain stem down your neck, clusters within your upper chest, continues down your torso, and clusters around your gut. That tension you feel in your chest when you're upset? That's related to your vagus. That pain in your gut when you're stressed? That's related to your vagus too. Your vagal tone directly affects the functioning of your heart, lungs, and digestion; that's a big empire to rule. It's the longest nerve in your entire nervous system, and nearly 90 percent of its communication is *from* your body, up *to* your brain; that is a lot of length for clustering—and a huge facility for generating the stress- or ease-related telegrams that I mentioned in chapter 3.

> How can we aid our system in finding balance when it seems to get so easily stuck on full throttle? Breathing can get the process started.

Your sympathetic branch is the gas pedal; your parasympathetic branch is the brake pedal. Stress can cause your system to put the pedal to the metal—of course, this is in an attempt to drive you toward safety (but it can also drive you up a wall). And with a robust gas pedal, we need a good braking system as well. After an auto-acceleration, breathing is probably the fastest and most direct brake we can apply. Scientifically speaking, the brake we are applying with our breathing is the *vagal brake.*

Recall the lioness I described in chapter 3, who successfully fled or fought her way to safety and then took time to circle in the grass, yawn, and lie down: that's a healthy use of gas pedal and brake pedal in balance. From the running to the resting, this animal's responses show a whole and healthy arc from sympathetic activity to parasympathetic activity. The lioness assessed danger; ran for her life; assessed newfound safety; and then rested, recalibrated, and *recovered*. How can we aid our system in finding such balance when it seems to get so easily stuck on full throttle? Breathing can get the process started.

But not just any breathing. We need rhythmic breathing. Porges (2014) explains that breathing in rapidly switches your body into sympathetic mode and prepares you for fight and flight. In contrast, extending your exhales and slowing your breathing rate switches your physiology into parasympathetic mode, to rest, digest, and just be. Your parasympathetic activity is hugely influenced by your vagus nerve, and your vagus nerve is hugely influenced by your breathing.

BALANCE WITHIN THE SYSTEM

The functioning of the sympathetic and parasympathetic could be likened to driving with *two* feet. In this analogy, you would have a foot on the brake *and* a foot on the gas, instead of the typical way we drive moving one foot *between* the brake and the gas. With this way of driving, it's a fine-tuning of both, not one or the other. There is a risk of letting one foot take a vacation while the other takes over. All gas, you get panic attacks; all brake, you pass out. It's also possible to press too hard on both pedals simultaneously, which can contribute to a system-wide reaction like chronic fatigue. The good news is, there is a balance of brake and gas taking place inside all of us all the time, and we have some access to that balance in each cycle of our breath.

Each inhale is a slight press on the gas: subtle heart rate increase, slight bronchial expansion within the lungs, and we become a little more alert. Each exhale is a slight press on the brake: subtle decrease in our heart rate, slight bronchial constriction in the lungs, and a little more relaxed. Rhythmic and balanced breathing facilitates just the right amount of each—a little gas on the inhale and a little brake on the exhale—no hectic turbo boosting, no melting brake pads.

BALANCING YOUR BREATH

Sucking in gulps of air over and over allows the gas foot to take over and speed you straight toward Stressville. Barely breathing at all presses way too hard on your braking foot and can stop you in your tracks. Both of these breathing reactions are common when stress takes over. Repeated gasps happen for many folks in anxiety-provoking situations, and the *incomplete exhales* that these gasps cause takes your foot right off of your brake. Holding your breath can go unnoticed until you begin to feel like your feet are stuck in setting cement, and your *incomplete inhales* can signal a slow but steady shutdown reaction. We've got to reacquaint ourselves with *complete* inhales and exhales, and recalibrate our gas and braking systems. Later in this chapter, we will learn how to use the breath to drive through high-stress obstacle courses, but before we do that, we have to learn how to just cruise across town.

Slow and Low

For cruising mode breathing, we develop "slow and low" breath cycles. This happens with a long, relaxed, and easy breath in. Followed by a slow, soothing, and complete breath out. Slow and low rhythmical breathing reacquaints you with your own breath during relaxing events— or non-events. The important thing is to learn and strengthen slow and low breathing in calm or neutral circumstances when stress activation is *not* present.

Slow and low breathing practice emphasizes finding your own natural breathing rhythm. To discover your own natural rhythm, it helps to relax as much as possible, especially the areas of your body around your lungs, like your belly and chest. The focus is on filling and emptying your lungs with the corresponding movement of your diaphragm pushing your belly out and drawing it in again. No intentional sucking in or tightening the abs during this kind of breathing. The less tension, the better. The more relaxed your belly is, the more freely your diaphragm can move, the fuller and more stress-relieving your breaths can be. Amazingly, slow and low rhythmic breathing can have a significant impact on your body-mind system—later, we'll take a look into some scientific studies.

Let's take time for a breathing break now. No time like the present. Any encounter with slow and low full inhales and exhales is a benefit to your brake, gas pedal, and entire vagus.

Breathing Break

1. Let your belly relax.

2. Allow your inhale to be slow and low in your belly

3. Give the breath time and room to gradually puff up your entire torso

4. Enjoy your breath in, no rush, and no strain

5. When you feel ready to breathe out, let the air smoothly release

6. Gradually and fully deflate your torso and gently draw your belly in to empty the lung fully

7. Repeat for the next few breaths. Easy. Relaxed. No strain. Good for you!

Now notice how you feel. How is your body right now? Are there any areas that feel at ease? If yes, notice those. Take them in. Let your self have that feeling for a moment. If not, are there any areas that are simply okay? Okay is plenty good enough for this practice. Give yourself a few moments to feel any okay parts of you, and notice if your breath can become like an assistant for you, helping you to navigate toward relief and ease. Helping you feel the safety and okayness you need and deserve.

Try adding in a few "ahhhhhhhs" or "hmmmmmms," long sighs or "om" type sounds. These add an extra vagal massage to your exhales. The longer the sound, the better; see if you can extend the sound for your entire exhale. "Ahhhhhhs" or "hmmmmmms" or "ooommmmmms" can be done anytime to wake up the vagus and send lots of telegrams of okayness from your belly to your brain!

(I like to do this in the car. I have lots of giggles ahhhh-ing and ooommm-ing as I cruse along...and to all the cars nearby, it just looks like I'm really into my favorite song.)

Relaxed slow and low breathing can recalibrate your sympathetic and parasympathetic inputs if you've been stuck with a heavy foot on either the gas or the brake—sometimes the lead foot lasts for days, weeks, months, or even years. On the surface, rhythmic breaths in and out are reminding your system how to access full breaths, but deep within you, your nervous system is learning the essential skill of oscillation—how to recover from, instead of getting stuck in the ups and downs of day-to-day life. With regular practice, the bridge between the breath in and breath out is well established, and your bridge between activation and recovery can become equally well established.

After repairs of this bridge, there is a progression to what I call "rescue breathing."

Rescue Breathing

In contrast to slow and low breathing practice—which is practiced when things are generally calm—rescue breathing is practiced when stress *is* present, during the actual event, in the throes of reactivity. It's meant to rescue you from driving headlong into a complete freak-out. If you find yourself about to lay on the gas, burn rubber, and fly into a panic, rescue breathing is a brief moment to lift your foot off the gas a bit—replacing jagged breathing with smooth breaths—while you also apply the brake, slowly and steadily, with each long exhale. On the other hand, if your stress has you slamming on the brakes and starting to stall, maybe beginning to go numb, rescue breathing will help you ease up on the brake—with robust inhales—and give you a little more oomph for the situation at hand. No need to figure out which state you're in and how to choreograph your breath. The intelligence of your body does that for you. Just a few long easy breaths in and out can jump-start your regulation, getting you back on track.

Max and I had been working on breathing skills for a few weeks when he told me this story. After becoming comfortable with rhythmic breathing practice, he began to use rescue breathing throughout his week during moments of stress. Common stressors for Max were presentations at work. He often felt too much pressure and too much scrutiny and was very tense during those meetings. As he approached one such presentation, he felt his chest tightening, his breathing becoming jagged, and his heart racing—too much gas pedal. He took a moment outside the conference room door for a few rescue breaths, intentionally softening his abdomen, encouraging slow and low breaths to move in and out. Just three or four breaths was all he took, and that is often all that's needed to shift a little away from full steam ahead and toward a slightly more comfortable cruising speed. He went into the boardroom feeling much less activated than he was used to, and he kept breathing throughout the meeting (as humans do), but this time, his breaths were more even and full. He left that meeting feeling far less stressed than usual and really proud of how well the presentation went.

We Need Both

To support our stress resilience, we will take these two approaches, establishing rhythmic breathing when things are pretty calm, cool, and collected, and integrating rescue breathing into moments that are—not so calm. First, we need to prepare ourselves for balanced pedal usage with slow and low breathing practice. You can practice in any free and unpressured moments you have: while stopped at a traffic light, during commercials, while you make dinner, before falling asleep at night, or before you get out of bed in the morning. Next, we'll learn how to round up our own personal first-responders team with rescue breathing. When things are not feeling so peachy, the rescue team of your breath can help to make the immediate circumstances seem a little safer. Rescue breathing happens in the midst of it all, at ground zero—getting by with a little help from our friends, our breaths in and breaths out.

Breathing is its own practice in this chapter; however, it is important to note that breathing is not enough on its own to deeply alter your system-wide stress reactivity. Corrective breathing practice lays the foundation, but it's not the whole enchilada. Your breath, with its direct influence on your vagus, will become an *aid* to each tool you'll learn in this book and *part* of each recovery from the stress imprints you long to be free from. *Combining* breathing with the other tools in these pages is what is needed to transform your body-mind system, bring balance to your nervous system, and build powerful paths of stress resilience.

Some Positive Side Effects May Include...

You know those TV ad warnings: "Negative side effects may include," and then a friendly sounding voice quickly rattles off a bunch of horrendous possibilities, which can include things like diarrhea or hair loss? Here I'd like to share some potential *positive* side effects of slow and low breathing (happily, none of them are loose bowels or thinning hair).

It may be inspiring to you, as it was to me, that regulated breathing has been linked to some pretty incredible health markers. Slow and low breathing has been shown to *reduce* inflammation throughout the body. Inflammation is believed to be a factor in migraines, chronic fatigue, irritable bowels, eczema—slow and low reduces chances of all those, and much more. Rhythmical breathing has also been recognized as a factor in overall health. People with regulated breathing live longer, healthier lives; they have stronger immune systems and even stronger hearts (Lehrer and Gevirtz 2014). The news about the power of our breathing is just so good, I hope it motivates you as it does me. I'll get into more research in a later section.

For ease of remembering, here is a helpful reminder for your tool kit. Consider this like the quick and short instructions that come with a favorite toy, device, project, or self-assembly furniture (no, wait; that's stress *increasing;* scratch that last one). This a quick guide to get you in the right direction. With time, this becomes internally directed—your body remembers it knows the way.

Relax your belly.

Everything else can wait a minute.

Slow and low breaths in and out.

Take your time; no rush.

Ancient Roots

Calming and soothing one's system with the breath is actually nothing new. While it is clear that recent scientific research supports the value of rhythmical breathing, this practice also has very ancient roots. Intentional breathing is said to have been central in yogic traditions dating back some five thousand years, and of course they've been Om-ing all that time as well. I used to think the Om was just a nice way to begin or end a class; now I know there is much more happening than that.

My initial introduction to slow and low breathing happened when I was nineteen. It was inside a bohemian light-filled loft in San Francisco that I feel lucky to have found during a period of extreme struggle. Among other issues, the breath helped me grapple with a huge grief surrounding the recent death of a dear family member. The breath became a trusted ally for me in times of stress. But much to my surprise, when my stress levels really soared, and my dysregulation was systematic, I seemed to forget how to breathe. I thought I already had this tool dialed, but it seemed that stress had deleted it from my contacts. When, two decades later, I started to study the research on rhythmical breathing, I was convinced that I needed to invest time in this simple yet profound practice once again. And luckily, none of us needs any special yoga training (or a bohemian loft in a big city) to breathe fully. Your lungs and awareness are the only prerequisites.

EVOLUTIONARY THEORY

If rhythmical breathing is so good for us and makes our bodies so happy, why do we react to stress with labored breathing—especially when it only makes the moment more laborious? When we assess stresses or threats, either consciously or below our consciousness, evolution has us either spring into action and take care of things with fighting or fleeing or duck and cover and wait for the problem to pass—a.k.a. freeze or shut down. Both of these automatically alter our breathing, heart rate, and blood pressure. We're just wired that way. And the wiring of course came from thousands of years of trial and error. You know—the slackers who kept kicking back, hum de ho, without so much as a [nose] hair out of place, were basically contentedly lounging on *le grande* dinner plate when the tigers arrived, while the survivors were hyperventilating and getting the flock out of there. Back then it made sense that when fight or flight was necessary, our breathing rate would quicken along with our heart. This would send oxygen and blood to the large muscles so they had the strength and energy to take care of business.

Ancient survivors were so clever that they also had option B, freezing or shutting down, if taking care of business was not possible and they needed to lay low and wait things out. With freeze and shutdown, their breathing would have become very slow and sporadic so they could wait as long as needed for the problem to clear out, breathing just enough to stay alive, but not enough to get noticed. To facilitate this long wait, their body would systematically close down all its internal factories as they became somewhat numb and mentally vacant. Think of a lizard standing statue still, barely inhaling and exhaling, waiting for long periods of time for your housecat to leave it alone so that it can get the heck out of there! And then there is option C, wherein both of these reactions happened simultaneously and they were gasping and barely breathing at the same time. In these cases, their system was simultaneously pulled toward both action and shutdown (and that's a party of a very special kind all its own).

Whether pulled toward action, inaction, or both at the same time, evolution causes our breathing to be dramatically compromised by stress. Back when stress meant we had to run from tigers, hyperventilating was adaptive. Now we hyperventilate while we're trying to give a public talk, take a test, or find an out-of-the-way restaurant. In these cases, rather than helping us to safety, our rapid breathing is just getting in the way. And of course, once upon a time an automatic duck-and-cover reaction was lifesaving, but now, not so much. Many of us struggle to keep ourselves from involuntarily vacating our own premises when stress is intensifying—and we find ourselves shutting down when we're just listening to the news, filling out tax forms, or trying to talk to a supervisor. It can feel like you're calling to yourself down a long dark tunnel—"Come back!"—but nothing is replying to you except your own echo. Breaking these maladaptive breathing patterns is an important step in the right direction.

Here we have a chance to use our evolved smarts to reroute these antiquated habits and instead breathe consciously, rhythmically, and in an oh-so-modern way.

SOME SCIENCE OF BREATHING

In the last decade or so, science has taken a keen interest in how widespread the effects of rhythmical breathing can be—widespread throughout your body, that is. Strong data show that breathing is an aid to recalibrating your sympathetic and parasympathetic activation and resetting your baseline. Before we dive into the science behind this tool, a breathing break for your breathing brake.

Breathing Break

Invite your belly to relax. Then allow your next few breaths to be slow and low. Give the breath time and room to gradually puff up your torso and then gradually deflate your torso. Repeat a few times. Add in some long "ahhhh-hhs" if it feels right. Good for you!

Rhythmical breathing is amazing for our physical health; it's a gift to our emotional well-being too. There is an abundance of scientific research on the topic. Rhythmical breathing is an easy way to quickly affect heart rate variability (HRV). As I mentioned earlier, on each inhale, our heart rate increases and on each exhale, it decreases. There is variability between the higher heart rate of an inhale and the lower heart rate of an exhale. In comes scientific enthusiasm for this variability and you have the HRV measure. High HRV means a wide range between the heart rate on inhale and the heart rate on exhale. Low HRV means a narrower range between these heart rates.

According to correlations found in numerous studies, high HRV is healthy; low HRV, not as healthy. For example, if a person is breathing shallow and quick breaths, their heart rate will increase just a little on a quick breath in and decrease just a bit on a curtailed breath out. This kind of breathing would generate a low HRV reading, indicating that that person is not so healthy. In contrast, if you take in a nice long breath that lasts a few seconds—maybe to a count of 5 or 6—your heart rate has ample time to increase. Then you follow this inhale with a nice long exhale that also lasts several seconds—ideally the same length as in the inhale—and your heart rate has plenty of time to drop again. With this kind of slow and low breathing, the variability between these two heart rates would be strong; it would be measured as high HRV, and you would be considered pretty healthy. High HRV is really good for the whole body-mind. Let's take a general look at some studies that examine this.

High HRV has been shown to increase parasympathetic engagement and vagal tone—rest, digest, tend, befriend (Prinsloo et al. 2011; Wells et al. 2012). High HRV was shown to relate to positive moods (Schwerdtfeger and Gerteis 2014). It can lead to lower anxiety levels and traumatic stress reactivity. HRV training has also been shown to decrease depressive symptoms (Karavidas et al. 2007). It has been found to be successful in reducing tension, fatigue, and anger (Lagos et al. 2008). High HRV can also lessen anxiety-related rumination and worry (Sherlin, Muench, and Wyckoff 2010). Not bad, eh? Now we'll dive into some specifics.

Study #1

In a 2009 study with Zucker and colleagues, thirty-eight participants with PTSD symptoms were selected from a substance use disorder clinic, and two groups of nineteen were formed. One group, the HRV group, was given a hand-held rhythmical breathing training device; the other, the PMR group, was given a guided CD for progressive muscle relaxation. Both groups were asked to spend twenty minutes a day for four weeks practicing either HRV or PMR. The compliance with the daily practice was mixed for both groups but did not seem to significantly affect the data.

Rhythmical breathing was impressive in reducing depression and also showed positive trends for bringing down PTSD symptoms. The compelling results for easing depression showed that, using the Beck depression inventory, 94 percent of the HRV group members were less depressed after the breathing practices, whereas only 58 percent of the PMR group members were less depressed after the muscle relaxation practices. Comparing the before-and-after results for symptoms associated with PTSD, using the PTSD symptom checklist, the HRV group again showed consistently better results than the PMR group. The HRV group decreased their PTSD symptoms by 27 percent, the PMR group by 18 percent. And not surprisingly, after the four-week practice period, the breath-training group had better HRV when at rest—that is, when *not* intentionally rhythmically breathing—than the muscle relaxation group, showing that rhythmic breathing practice has a lasting positive effect.

Study #2

A study with ninety-five college students conducted by Steffen and colleagues in 2017 assessed the quality of the participants' mood before and after rhythmic breathing. There were four groups in the study, intentionally breathing in different ways as instructed:

- Subjects slightly overbreathing—a little too fast

- Subjects slightly underbreathing—a little too slow

- Subjects breathing rhythmically and comfortably—kind of like Goldilocks and the three bears, "just right"

- Control subjects just quietly resting with their eyes open, not directing their breathing at all

The experiment consisted of the subjects breathing for 15 minutes—or sitting calmly, for the control group—then filling out surveys on their mood and stress level. They then took a math test meant to stress them a little, followed by resting for ten minutes, then making a final report of their mood and stress level. In terms of stress and mood, the only subjects whose mood improved after the breathing practice were the ones in the comfortable rhythmic breathing group. This group also had better HRV than the other three groups. Again, this shows that slow and low *comfortable breathing,* as opposed to too slow or too fast, links to better mood and better HRV.

Study #3

Professional musicians were selected for a 2012 study because of their high incidence of preperformance anxiety and post-performance depression. Wells and colleagues (2012) divided forty-six musicians ages nineteen through forty-six into three groups: two breathing groups and one control group. Breathing group A was given basic low and slow breathing instructions *and* connected to a computer for feedback intended to maximize their unique breathing rhythm or resonant frequency over a thirty-minute period. Breathing group B was also given slow and low breathing instruction but *not* connected to a computer for feedback, using their own awareness as their guide for thirty minutes. Group C was told to read any material of their choice for thirty minutes.

After assessing their baseline measures, each group was intentionally provoked by being instructed that they had five minutes to study their music and would then be recorded on video; they were to play to the best of their abilities without stopping if they made a mistake. They were told their recorded performance would be evaluated for accuracy and musical interpretation. They then engaged in the previous breathing or reading for thirty minutes, then had their anxiety and emotional reactivity measured.

The study showed an increase in vagal brake functioning for both of the breathing groups and decreased vagal brake functioning for the reading group. The results also demonstrate that the anxious members of breathing groups experienced decreased anxiety symptoms after the breathing session while the anxious members of the reading group experienced anxiety increase. Breathing was consistently better at eliciting a parasympathetic response, which the researchers described as leading to a focus on enjoying the performance, whereas the reading group tended to focus on their mistakes and possible failures. Importantly, there was *not* a noticeable benefit for the group that received computer feedback of their breathing versus those participants who self-directed their slow and low breathing. Good news for those of us who do not have a breath monitoring system already installed on our home computers.

Subtle and Profound Effects

What might this look like in your life? How might this help you with your stress? It will be different for everyone. The contribution that your breathing makes to your life comes in a variety of forms.

Try This: Notice Your Breath and Stress Connection

How linked are breathing and stress for you?

1. When I'm stressed, changes in my breathing are:

    a. Very pronounced _____   b. Subtle _____   c. Not noticeable _____

2. I sometimes catch myself:

    a. Panting _____   b. Holding my breath _____   c. Neither _____

3. I feel like I can't take a full and deep breath:

    a. Often _____   b. Sometimes _____   c. Never _____

4. When I'm stressed I feel light-headed or dizzy:

    a. Often _____   b. Sometimes _____   c. Never _____

5. When I'm stressed I can feel my belly or chest tighten making it hard to breathe

    a. Often _____   b. Sometimes _____   c. Never _____

Take note of how many of your answers are "a"s. Four or five "a"s indicates your breathing and stress are fairly linked; four or five "b"s indicates your breathing and stress are moderately linked; four or five "c"s indicates your breathing and stress are not very linked. A combination—say, two or three each "a"s and "b"s, "a"s and "c"s, or "b"s and "c"s—indicates that sometimes your breath is part of your stress reaction, sometimes not.

This is not a static result; it may—and is likely to—change over time. Your awareness of your breathing may also change. Because of both of these factors, you might want to answer these questions again in a month or two after you've increased your awareness of your breathing overall.

No judgment needed: it is not better to have "a"s or better to have "c"s. This is just your body talking to you, letting you know whether the breath is one of its primary stress expressions or not.

For Susan, the woman I described at the start of this chapter, her struggle with gasping and shortness of breath was a substantial contributor to her stress. Not getting enough air played a big role in her stress reaction, and the experience of full breaths was a significant aid to her stress resilience. For others it is subtler—like for Max, who used slow and low and rescue breaths as a reassuring background support throughout his stress recovery. And sometimes, breathing starts in the background and then moves very surely to the forefront. For my client Viola, her breathing helped little by little over time and then one day was profoundly impactful.

Over decades, Viola's emotional overwhelm and pain had become lodged in her body, becoming physical overwhelm and pain. She had been struggling with a few autoimmune diseases and was so tired of feeling so tired all the time. The breath became an important ally for Viola.

First, she adopted a regular awareness practice that included slow and low breathing. Reclining in the comfort of her home, she would take time to breathe and be. This created a *positive* imprint and a new pathway of regulated breathing that I saw her use many times in our work together.

As a result of Viola's regular breathing practice, whenever I asked her to sense her body during our sessions together, a few deep breaths accompanied the process. One day, as she sensed into her body with the sensations of the breath there as a trusted companion to her process, she described feeling a lightening that hadn't been there for a long time. With the help of her easy breathing, she stayed with her sensations to witness them change and morph from her familiar fatigue to an uprightness and strength she hadn't felt in a while. Still breathing slow and low, she placed her awareness on her uprightness, her breath helping her to take in this big shift. This was, of course, just one step in a series of steps that helped her lessen her chronic fatigue, which can be a complex and deeply embedded stress response. But I've seen again and again that the breath can be a helpful aid in being with our bodies as they transform and heal. Whatever it is you are facing, why not add a little more breath to the situation?

HOW YOU CAN BREATHE WITH AND THROUGH STRESS

The first *how* is to relax, trust your body, and remember you've been breathing all your life. It's important that our stress-reducing practices do not actually become stress increasing.! To that end, I recommend that you practice whenever and wherever you can. For example, you don't need to practice your breathing all on its own to the exclusion of other things. After all, we breathe while simultaneously doing other things all day long. Yes, you may need to give yourself a little time to get the hang of it, but this is not a pass-fail task. You are simply improving something you are already fairly good at—if you weren't *good enough*, you wouldn't be alive. I think you'll find that the breath can become an enjoyable companion. You can hang out with it while you drive to work, send emails, grocery shop, take out the trash...and my personal favorite: while waking up in the morning and falling asleep at night.

First Step: Rhythmic Breathing to Balance Your Nervous System

The first key is to undo the constriction around your lungs and diaphragm that stress can create. The opposite of contracting is relaxing. You may be surprised to feel that just by relaxing your belly, your breath will noticeably move more deeply into your lungs. Add to that a little attention to filling up the ribcage and chest areas as well, and you will have taken a very full breath. It is helpful to have your torso somewhat elongated too—it's hard to breathe fully when you're crunched, cramped, or significantly slouched. But there is no need to take any of this to an extreme. Easy does it. Straining doesn't help; it might even lead to over-breathing. There is a happy medium between too much and too little. The middle ground we're looking for should feel comfortable and fairly easy. Use your sensations as a guide.

Many scientific studies have found that approximately six breaths per minute is a good average for optimal adult slow and low breathing rhythm. But there is no need to break out a stopwatch every time you want to take a breathing break. If glancing at a clock a few times as you get used to this practices helps you, great. If the numbers, or clocks, or time frames are creating stress, this is important information. Listen to it. I encourage you to leave out any details of this practice that lead you to feel there is a good and a bad way to breathe—that is *not* what we are going for here.

If you experience any stress or strain when trying out slow and low breathing, it can help to focus on just your exhale and just let the inhale happen. Think of this as a gentle, no-expectation nudge to yourself to focus on breathing out fully, then relaxing, softening your belly and allowing the next breath in to just happen.

Because you've emptied your lungs so completely with your conscious exhale, your next intake of breath will automatically be more full. Follow that nice long inhale by another full exhale, emptying the lungs as much as possible, then again relax your belly and allow another full breath in. Now you are well on your way to rhythmic breathing!

> Remember two things:
> - This is meant to relieve stress, not create it.
> - You already breathe in and out fairly well all day long.

Try This: Rhythmical Breathing

1. Relax and get comfortable wherever you are sitting, standing, or lying down.

2. Soften your belly and chest, letting tension go from your torso.

3. Notice your breathing for a few breath cycles. In, out, in, out.

4. Then with a soft belly, invite your next breath in to be slow, low, and long.

5. Without any rush, let your breath out be long and complete, with a little attention to squeezing out your lungs like a sponge by slightly engaging your abdominal muscles.

6. Then intentionally soften your belly muscles and again invite a long breath in, filling your belly and chest.

7. Again, a full breath out, emphasizing emptying the lungs.

8. No rush; take all the time you need, and be sure that your breathing is comfortable. There should be no strain here, just relaxed long breaths.

Second Step: Rescue Breathing

Once you've become familiar with rhythmic breathing and your body has developed a bridge between sympathetic activation and parasympathetic activation (remember, each inhale slightly engages your nervous system and each exhale slightly soothes it), you can learn to use this bridge for a quick rescue. You can use it like a getaway route from Stressville. Because, as I've said, when we are stressed, we often involuntarily stop breathing fully; with rescue breathing, we bring a little "voluntarily" into the situation. You can take a few moments to decrease your reactivity with a few slow and low breaths instead of increasing your body's stress reactivity with erratic breathing. The next time you find yourself heading straight toward Stressville, try taking a few rescue breaths and see if you can release any of the pressure that had been building up.

Try This: Rescue Breathing

1. While in the midst of life's stressors, as you notice your body going into a stress reaction, begin to intentionally direct your breathing.

2. Start by relaxing your belly and chest as much as you are able to— even if it is just a little. Every little bit of ease helps!

3. Then focus on guiding your next breath *out*. Try to fully exhale, use your abdominal muscles to press the air out of your lungs.

4. Allow your next inhale to be full. Your body will naturally want to take a full breath in after that long breath out you just had. Try to relax and allow your body time for this inhale.

5. Repeat the next full exhale, guiding all the air out of your lungs.

6. Again, allow your body to drink in its next breath, filling your lungs with a fresh breath of air.

These breaths can shift you away from being derailed by stress reactivity and head you toward feeling like you can stay the course. You're not going to suddenly feel like dancing in the streets, so don't feel like you've done anything wrong if that doesn't happen. This is a gentle nudge toward regulation; about slightly turning down the volume of the stress messages traveling between your body and brain, and slightly turning up the volume of the "you can handle this" messages that are roaming around in your body-mind system.

In the course of this chapter, I hope you've developed an enhanced relationship with your breath and it has become a trusted companion. In the next chapter, we'll progress from breathing to seeing.

CHAPTER 5

Seeing and Sensing
Here and Now

Now we're going to take a look at what happens to our perspective when stress is part of the situation. Again, there will be guidance for you to experience this firsthand, as well as some of the grounded evidence behind this tool. Body to brain, brain back to body, and around again; deepening your connection to both body and mind and ultimately connecting them as one.

WHY WE NEED A CLEAR VIEW

I was standing in the grocery store, rushing to check out and get to an important appointment I was late for—an appointment that carried some pressure for me and that I somewhat dreaded. That's when I saw, out of the corner of my eye, someone entering the store; someone I was, shall we say, not prepared to talk with just then. This was activating for me for many reasons: rushing, lateness, and the importance of the appointment were the setup for my stress mountain to begin to feel like a dormant volcano might well erupt again. The lava began to bubble as this particular someone walked in my direction. These were all known stress triggers for me, so it wasn't a total surprise, but it wasn't comfortable when I felt my heart rate quicken, my mouth go dry, and sweat prick at my upper lip and underarms. As I tried to steady myself, I observed my perceptions shifting. The market *seemed* to be transforming from a welcoming or at least neutral space into a somewhat hostile environment. Then, without any conscious direction from me, my eyes guided themselves to the large windows at the front. With this simple action, my whole body-mind system began to slowly but surely shift.

It was autumn, and the fall colors were particularly beautiful—something I always appreciate seeing. As I gazed at and enjoyed the reddening leaves, I felt my heart rate begin to slow—a very welcome relief. I took very intentional notice of this relief for a few moments. Then I brought my attention back to the leaves and surrounding skyline, noticing my body temperature dropping. I felt a slight swell of gladness as I finished checking out sans the unwanted conversation. I let this too sink in as I walked out into the crisp air, saw the sunlight through the tree branches, and viscerally tracked my return to regulation.

This was a little blip of stress in the larger scheme of things, but celebrating small gains in self-regulation is extremely important for building the resilience we'll need for larger stresses and even for the whoppers. On that particular day I realized that, much to my surprise and pleasure, my practices of seeing and sensing had become a habit, so much so that my system just reached for the tool and used it for my benefit before I even really knew resilience pathway maintenance had begun.

This is what I want for you—tools at the ready, able to help with life's ups and downs. Tool #2 centers on seeing and sensing, because what we see and sense intimately affects how we feel. After we have become thrown off balance, or feel turned upside-down, it is so important that we have tools to right ourselves again. Tool #2 offers a simple way to reorient, one that ushers you back from Stressville and into here and now.

> Celebrating small gains in your ability to self-regulate is a big help in building strong resilience pathways.

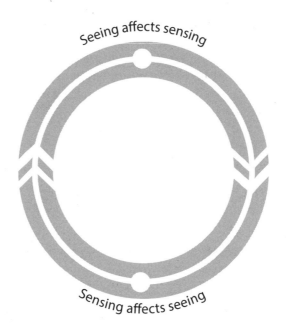

Seeing affects sensing

Sensing affects seeing

Try This: Basic Seeing and Sensing

1. Invite your eyes to look freely around the place you are right now. Explore the area visually, looking up, down, and side to side.

2. Let your eyes find something they enjoy looking at. It can be anything—a picture on a wall, a view out of a window, the color of the ceiling, a shadow on the floor.

3. As you allow your eyes to rest there, just take in the view. Light and easy.

4. Now notice what it feels like in your body as you rest your gaze on this pleasing view.

5. Pay particular attention to areas that feel at ease or less tense than other areas.

6. Stay with that for a moment.

7. Now let your gaze soften even more and attend to your sensations again. Has the area of ease grown or expanded to other parts of your body?

8.   Sense any parts of you that are less tense, even by degrees. Notice your easeful parts all together. Take a few breaths. Enjoy.

End this exercise whenever you feel complete. A few seconds or a few moments; no need to stay any longer than you would like to. Good for you!

CRUCIAL CONVERSATIONS

There is an essential conversation taking place between your body and mind about what you are seeing in the world *around* you and what you are sensing in the world *within* you. This body-mind conversation can be a fairly accurate account or a very falsified rendition of what's going on. And if you do not have a clear enough view and a safe enough place within to rest, this conversation can get out of hand.

When we are stressed, fearful, overwhelmed, angry, and the like, the conversation ceases to be a neutrally reported news update between our body and brain and becomes more like a hastily written mean tweet, replete with lots of ALL CAPS and!!!! exclamations. And of course, as is the case with hastily written mean tweets, the truth and reliability of these news flashes are pixel-thin. They also cause us trouble because they are, well, alarming.

When our mind-body conversation is dominated with alarming and stressful stuff, our view of the world is obscured; we just do not see reality clearly. When our body begins to feel extreme stress, our survival brain zeros in on the stress stuff that's happening, and unfortunately also makes up stress stuff that's *not* happening—but our fear brain believes it is real. Adding insult to injury, that stressful stuff we zero in on—real or imagined—makes us *more* stressed. Also, when seeing and sensing are compromised, the *nonstress* stuff of our world gets very little of our attention. And when stress is exceptionally high, we can miss the nonstress stuff entirely—even when it's right in front of us. In high stress, we actually do not see the nonstress.

When the volume has been turned up way too high on the stress stuff, and there is a mute on the nonstress stuff, simple acts of seeing and sensing can bring us back to reality and offer relief to our body-mind system.

There's another obstacle to this crucial body-mind conversation: our stress brain has *no* time awareness. When our stress brain is activated and we are in fight, flight, or freeze, as far as the stress brain is concerned, the stress of today and the stress of yesterday are both happening *now*. In

> Seeing is not always believing when high-level stress is involved.

these instances, our body acts like yesterday's stress is now, today's stress is now, tomorrow's potential stress is now, and all that activation becomes part of now.

Take, for example, a car accident survivor. Their muscles constrict and their heart rate leaps while they are simply making a left turn; their body-mind is responding to being behind the wheel today as if that long-ago accident were happening now. This also happens with smaller stresses, like seeing an adversary across the room at a party and feeling as though the ongoing battles the two of you had months ago have just reoccurred in the moment your eyes meet. Or even subtler still, the sight of the restaurant that gave you food poisoning a few years ago, yet it still makes you feel nauseous. Seeing and sensing can pull the stress brain out of yesterday and bring you back to here and now.

FROM IN TO OUT AND OUT TO IN

Stressed humans can become prone to tunnel vision and confuse yesterday with today. This then raises the question: are we accurately seeing and sensing our external and internal landscapes? In the mid-1960s and early 1970s, psychologists James J. Gibson and Richard L. Gregory debated whether perception happens from our eyes to our thoughts or from our thoughts to our eyes. To expand: do we see what is actually happening around us with accurate vision and then think about it, or do our thoughts and memories interfere, *preceding* what our eyes take in, adding information to what our eyes are "seeing"?

The research bore out that it's both—depending on our stress levels. When we are feeling fairly safe and okay, we can more or less see and hear what is actually happening in front of us, then process it further through thinking: this is perceiving information from our *eyes* to our *thoughts*. In contrast, when we are feeling scared, stressed, or overwhelmed, our thoughts interject *before* our eyes can get the picture. Our mind begins to tell a story. The story our thoughts create is intended to corroborate our *feelings* of fear and stress. Without realizing it, we start "seeing" this story around us: this is perceiving from our *thoughts* to our *eyes*. Stress can substantially affect what we see, hear, and smell in our environment. In instances of intense stress, the internal landscape can alter our perceptions of the external landscape; your body might be doing the thinking for your mind.

Neuroception

As Levine, Porges, and van der Kolk all explain in their work, our body-mind systems are constantly assessing for safety and threat, which then prompts our survival brain to *automatically respond* to the sensory information we've received from our environment. These environmental impressions are then transmitted throughout our nervous system, becoming a *felt experience* of safety or threat. Porges calls this *neuroception.*

> Healthy neuroception can be a quiet ally for your body-mind, but stress-driven neuroception can be a hidden disrupter.

Neuroception is an automatic process, happening below your consciousness, of appraising and reacting to what you see, hear, smell, and feel happening around you, which then unconsciously and automatically determines what is happening within you. The reverse is also true, but more on that in a moment. In a regulated mind-body, our neuroception is more or less accurate. In a dysregulated system, our neuroception often tells tall tales. What's more, extreme and chronic stress often leads to persistently faulty neuroception, wherein we may see danger that isn't there, hear criticism that wasn't spoken, or feel persecuted by an innocent bystander.

Neuroception and Feedback Loops

With accurate neuroception, you can recognize a young man walking toward your door as a parcel delivery professional; you can see that he's carrying a small box. With faulty neuroception, you could very well see that delivery professional as an intruder. This "sighting" would then become a cue from your external landscape to create automatic reactions in your internal landscape. You might begin to inexplicably gasp for air or feel a knot in your stomach. This could then be followed by an adrenaline surge and surprising tension in your legs—biological preparation to fight or flee. You might even find yourself having a

...Around it goes, turning up the volume and intensity on your stress reactivity...

burst of anger at this trespasser—biological self-defense! Meanwhile, your fear-driven brain will be generating a narrative about this man and his intentions. The next lightning-speed reactions would be your fear-driven brain cueing your eyes to "see" a mean look in his eyes, "recognize" his overpowering stance, and "identify" his questionable intentions.

Cliff Notes to faulty neuroception: Bill suffers from extreme-stress imprints. Bill begins to feel anxious. He automatically and unconsciously scans his environment for danger. Bill "sees" the danger he has been scanning for. He feels more afraid. Bill's brain organizes a narrative to explain his physical fear. He "sees" the story his brain is creating. Bill is then, of course, more afraid. Sound familiar?

Many of us have been there time and time again. This becomes an ongoing *negative feedback loop*.

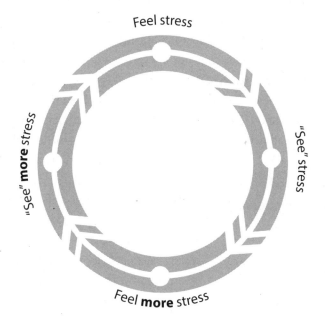

Feel stress

"See" stress

Feel **more** stress

"See **more** stress

Within this negative feedback loop, faulty seeing can spawn fear and create faulty sensing, but the opposite is also true. With neuroception, faulty sensing can also spawn faulty seeing and lead to—you guessed it—fear. In addition to the brain and sensing connections I describe in chapter 3, the brain has another sophisticated monitoring system specifically designated to track our sensations: the survival brain. Your survival brain is constantly tracking sensations and reacting to them well before your conscious brain has processed any thoughts on the matter. *Sensations* linked to stress, fear, and overwhelm can trigger a negative feedback loop as frequently as the "sightings" just described.

Neuroception and Your Brain

Recent advances in neuroscience have identified the neural circuits connected to our sensation monitoring system, and it is clear that this system can elicit a robust stress response. The front brain has an area that watches over you; van der Kolk called it the *watchtower*. This watcher or overseer is uniquely connected to your bodily sensation centers and very influenced by what you feel at any given moment.

What's more, this overseer has a direct line to the alarm system of the survival brain—the amygdala. While the overseer is located in the modern, more evolved part of the brain—the prefrontal cortex (PFC)—it communicates to the very primitive, stress-driven brain—the limbic brain and brainstem. This direct line means the sensation-aware regions of the modern brain can transmit alarming news to the primitive brain and quickly cause a ruckus. Yet these sensation centers can also swiftly share soothing news with the survival brain and help things hum along calmly. Seeing and feeling okayness should not be underestimated.

This is good news! The same circuitry that can startle and alarm us also has great connectivity for eliciting a soothing response. We can reemploy our circuitry, replacing its job of contributing to negative feedback loops, and instead direct our brain-body to use sensations to evoke *positive* feedback loops. This chapter will teach you how to enlist this help from your seeing and sensing abilities.

... around and around *this* goes until you've decreased your stress level, even by just a little. That is a good-enough start for this practice. We'll take it!

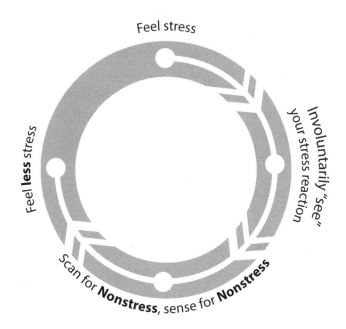

Somatic experts agree that this ongoing body-mind conversation takes place *first* through sensations and sensory impressions and *then* becomes thoughts and beliefs. Just as sensations and sense impressions are the basis of our *automatic* reactions to stress, they will also be the basis of our *intentional* response to stress.

SLOWING THINGS DOWN AND SEEING

Taking a look around can also give us a much-needed break from our stress. As I mentioned in chapter 2, when it comes to gaining stress resilience, less can be more. When our stress brain is activated, our entire body-mind system tends to speed up. While this produces the increase in heart rate and breathing we've covered previously, it also can mean that stress memories swoop down on us. As our body speeds up, so does our mind, and this speedy mind can take us into stress memory too fast and too far. To keep from diving too deeply into the stress pool, we can use seeing and sensing to slow things down.

My client Helen and I were working online, discussing a situation at her place of work. As she described the persecution she had been feeling from several of her colleagues at work, the term "harassment" came to her. Discussing this clearly increased her activation; with the activation, I could see a familiar blankness occurring behind her eyes. She was becoming less with me, less with herself, and more with her painful memories. When her activation levels headed too high, I gently interrupted her and asked her to take a look around—to let her eyes find something pleasing in her environment. Because she and I were working online, she was looking around her own home, which felt cozy and reassuring to her. As she glanced around the room, her gaze rested on a view out a window that pleased her. She took in this vista and noticed her breathing deepened. I asked her if she could allow and even enjoy those breaths. She told me the tension she had been feeling in her hands was lessening. We took a few moments for her to feel that process of tension releasing out of her body. I could see Helen becoming more behind her own eyes than she had been a few moments ago, when her system was being overcome with fight-or-flight reactivity. She became more *in herself* again too, more embodied. Seeing and sensing can be that quick, that affecting. Of course, it is not the only tool we need to heal habitual activation and wounds. Yet it can become quite a dependable aid for sudden bursts of activation.

> Just as sensations are the basis of our *automatic stress reactions*, they will also be the basis of our *intentional stress recoveries*.

Break Time

Read the instructions, then take this break.

Many little seeing and sensing breaks are great for our nervous systems.

1. Take a nice long look around. Gentle and slow. No rush.

2. Let your eyes find something they enjoy looking at. Maybe something in the room, or outside of it? A view? A shaft of light? Something on a wall? Perhaps even just a direction; looking down to the

right or up to the left, for example, might feel good for whatever reason.

3. Once you find that thing, view, or direction to rest your eyes on, just relax your gaze there. Maybe even your focus softens and blurs a bit; that's just fine too. No need to focus; let your eyes decide how they want to see.

4. Next, notice your body. What happens in your body as you rest your gaze on something pleasing? Can you sense your breath? What happens in your breathing when you rest your gaze and sense your body? Allow your breath to join in this seeing and sensing.

5. Now just take this experience in. Easy does it. Conclude whenever you feel done.

REPLACING NEGATIVE FEEDBACK LOOPS WITH POSITIVE ONES

For those of us who might self identify as high worriers or as prone to extreme stress, the world around us can at times appear to be an unwelcoming or overwhelming place. As I've described, when you are stressed, scared, or triggered, your thoughts can interrupt your seeing and convince your eyes of things that aren't actually there. This can all happen at lightning speed as the whole body-mind system revs up in response to stress activation. With brain as the seer, we're stuck unconsciously creating a point of view (pun intended) about the environment and then automatically scanning our surroundings for evidence that validates that point of view—entering right back into a negative feedback loop.

From within the negative feedback loop, we literally do not see or hear the evidence to the contrary—if left to our instincts alone. However, by teaching our system to reorient and reconnect with our here-and-now external and internal landscapes, we can *exit* these loops. Our false, fear-induced perceptions can be updated with a view of relative safety. And as self-regulation increases, the world appears and feels welcoming again.

With these perceptions of safety, we can enter the *positive* feedback loops that are also available to us.

NEGATIVE TO POSITIVE IN DAILY LIFE

Mary was walking into services one day at her synagogue. Her synagogue had become a source of stress after she experienced several undermining and demeaning interactions and events there. Standing before Mary in the greeting line was a person who had been particularly unkind to her some months before. She immediately felt her threat awareness heightening, which led her breathing to become strained and a knot to form in her stomach. She felt dizzy, and the room appeared full of antagonistic others.

With the skills of sensing and seeing, Mary was able to track what was happening in her body-mind and take some steps to soothe her system. She scanned the room to identify one safe person. She found one and let her gaze rest on this kind person across the room. As Mary took in this safe other, she felt her body unclench and her breathing spontaneously deepen. Because she was well-practiced with this tool, she knew it was important to take in these shifts toward ease and safety, no matter how large or small. As this seeing and sensing transpired, the room appeared less threatening to her and the people in it a bit kinder. As the evening went on, she was even able to enjoy a conversation with the safe person she had first identified.

Through intentionally using the tool of seeing safety and sensing safety, she brought herself back from fear and reactivity to relative comfort and degrees of increased well-being. This event began an important shift for Mary. Her synagogue transformed from a triggering and dysregulating environment to one that, over time and with continued somatic-regulation practices, she came to enjoy. Seeing and sensing was not the only tool she applied to her stress, but it was part of an effective collection.

> While our minds can and do fool us, coming back to clarity is possible.
>
> Seeing and sensing are part of the return.

Next time you find yourself in a stressful environment, maybe seeing hostile others, I encourage you to take a moment for seeing and sensing. See if it might turn the volume down on your stress just a bit.

SCIENCE OF SEEING AND SENSING

Nineteenth-century scientists revealed that our general reactivity and its repetitious nature are hardwired in us. In the 1870s, Darwin observed that human bodies *automatically* react to subtle stimuli from their environment; an environment that is perceived as safe engenders a functional, at-ease body, and an environment perceived as dangerous incites an activated, tense body.

Together with Pavlov's 1890s research on mammals' predisposition to *automatically repeat* physical responses with a cue, these findings identify an automatic feedback loop cycling through our bodies. Of course we all know about Pavlov's dogs that would predictably salivate with the sound of a bell, as they anticipated being fed. In early history, this might have looked like a cavewoman repeatedly hyperventilating at the site of a tiger, as she feared *becoming* lunch; today it could be regularly breaking into a sweat at the sight of an angry supervisor before we attend a team lunch. *Bam,* it just happens: our body and mind react (whether lunch is involved or not!). We're wired this way.

It has long been established in the scientific community that we humans have a bias toward recognizing and processing negative or threatening information in our environment, rather than the positive. While we all share an aptitude for tuning out the good and tuning in the bad, those of us who are prone to stress are even more likely to see the bad and miss the good.

Beginning in the 1970s, scientists speculated and then confirmed that anxious individuals were slower to recognize positive stimuli than their nonanxious counterparts (Mogg et al. 1993). More recently, Beard and Amir (2010) showed that anxious individuals interpreted ambiguous information in their environment as negative information, and their negative interpretations *increased* as their anxiety levels rose.

Study #1

This perspective has continued through 2017 with a study that compared "high worriers" to "low worriers" and their attention to threats in their environment. Goodwin and colleagues (2016) found that the high worriers were more attentive to threat cues than the low worriers. The high worriers reported that they could not cognitively control where their attention went; rather, threat attentiveness happened *automatically* for them. This underscores the top-down versus bottom-up argument from the chapter 4. This study indicates that we can't think our way through this negative feedback loop, we have to feel our way out of it.

Study #2

In a 2012 review of scientific literature by Hirsch and Mathews, it was explained that if a person has a repeated experience with a particular threat, she can create habitual responses to this *and similar* threat cues. This review concluded that because of our negative bias, ambiguous cues are easily misinterpreted as negative. When we identify threat cues in our environment that our stress brain is familiar with, this tends to cause an involuntary reaction that mimics our previous reactions to this type of threat. Even a cue with a shade of familiarity can kick the stress brain into full-blown reactivity.

For example, if Sue has been attacked by several dogs over the years and has lived through many episodes of dog reactivity, she may have an involuntary reaction to the sight of dogs. She may even automatically react to a dog in the distance. If this stress-brain reactivity is really ingrained, the mere mention of a friend's dog can ignite a surge of adrenaline, racing heart, difficulty breathing, or feeling like her legs are stuck in cement even as she wants desperately to run. This is an automatic reaction that originally begins with an actual perception of threat but can then progress to an array of "seeing" the threat.

We all live with our own stress cues. For some, it is the sight of an ex-husband; for others, a crosswalk; it can also be an empty room or a pile of bills. It helps to get to know your stress cues; I'll address this in more detail in chapter 6. However, most importantly, developing your new feedback loops, cycling from body to mind to body again, will change the way the cues affect you overall. It takes some time, but your body-mind system can heal. Seeing and sensing are supports in the process.

Study #3

In a 2017 study with twenty-two anxious participants and fourteen healthy volunteers, Grossi and his colleagues scanned participants' brains with an fMRI scanner, collecting fifty images of each brain. The study investigated whether interoception-related areas of the brain would light up on the scanner when subjects viewed their environment—specifically, reading facial expressions and body movements of other people. This would allow scientists to compare what's happening in the anxious to the nonanxious brain. Did anxious brains have as much sensation awareness as nonanxious brains?

The study confirmed that the people who were *not* anxious were really effective seers and sensers. Their brains were good at coordinated seeing and sensing. In contrast, the anxious individuals did not have this sensing and seeing coordination—meaning that those who were slow or clumsy with *sensing their own body* were in the anxious group. This study indicates that being connected to one's own *felt sense* is a component in anxiety reduction and stress resilience.

The Grossi study also revealed that sensing the *nonstressful* parts of your body quiets the "mean tweet" version of things. Other research has shown that nonstressful sensation awareness can deactivate neural fear centers. In this study, the brain scans of the *non*anxious folks showed hearty neural connections to their *non*stress sensations. In contrast, the anxious folks had strong neural connectivity to their *stress* sensations. When we attend primarily to our stress sensations, we're traveling a familiar yet unwanted route—destination: increased stress. Sensing our okay or even neutral sensations can put us back on course to well-being.

Studies #4 and #5

In a pair of studies conducted by Zotev, Young, and colleagues (Zotev et al. 2013; Young et al. 2014), nearly instantaneous self-regulation was possible for healthy participants. They uncovered a process in participants' successful and swift self-regulation: pacifying communication between the front brain, including sensation-aware areas, and the fear-driven amygdala in the primitive brain. By sending soothing messages from their sensation awareness to their stress center, those research volunteers were like self-regulating ninjas!

We can all become self-regulating ninjas. All of our brains are constantly changing and ready to be strengthened in new and improved ways. If healthy brains do their heavy lifting with sensing, let's all get in our brain workout—with sensing being one of our primary exercise circuits.

Break Time

Experiment with guiding yourself through a seeing and sensing exercise. Play with it, make it your own.

The basic idea is to see and feel the here and now.

If for any reason that feels uncomfortable, repeat either the exercise on page 95 or 102.

Enjoy. Good for you!

EVOLUTIONARY THEORY

Why do our brains do this? When we humans lived in much less secure spaces—on the plains, for example—we were incredibly vulnerable to our environment. To stay safe and, well, alive, we needed to be really cognizant of what was nearby at all times. The plains people who survived were excellent at scanning their environment and knowing what was afoot nearby. When actual threats did come into view or earshot, tenacious self-protectors needed to solely focus on the possible threat: *I see the tiger, coming from the east, I hear it crunching grass under its feet rather slowly, and conclude that it won't get to me for several minutes.* This was not a time to relax for a moment and take in the particularly beautiful sunset, or to enjoy the sound of a really lovely bird song up above. If that ancestor let herself be distracted by nonessentials like a sunset or a bird—or anything *not* having to do with the threat in her surroundings— she would be, to put it succinctly, a goner.

Here we are in our cozy homes and cars, with lockable doors, but our brains still function in much the same way. Our primitive brain has evolved to unconsciously—and nearly constantly—scan our environment to assess safety and threat. If something triggers us, from either the external or the internal landscape, we are wired to go on high alert and begin to see and hear everything we can about that threat. Simultaneously, we are wired to automatically tune out everything else, a.k.a. the *okay* stuff around us. Those of us with extreme stress imprints can too easily find ourselves involuntarily looping into feeling stress, seeing stress, tuning out all the nonstress, and then seeing and feeling more and more stress. It's like having only one song on your MP3 player—one track, on repeat.

Fast-forward to today: experts agree that those who have experienced extreme stress and trauma can become stuck in hypervigilance, a thousands-of-years-old solution to a very modern problem. With nervousness and stress running our mind-body system, internal unrest drives us to Stressville. And on the way, all our activation causes us to "identify" the threats that our stress brain thinks *must be* looming near us. In this state, we are on edge, blinded to reality; we can even have a hard time relaxing when we *are* safe. What worked to save our ancestors all those years ago isn't as well suited to today's world.

WHEN SEEING AND SENSING FOOLS US

Negative feedback loops can be tricky things. They can feel so real, seem so related to the situation at hand, when in reality they are anything but. Negative loops don't always relate to today; they can be sort of flown in from an unrelated circumstance. I explain to my clients that activation can be like a helicopter seeking a landing pad; dysregulation might be floating around inside of us, look for a situation to drop down into. A cue can pop up with just a whiff of trigger and our body-mind can hop on the stress train.

Here's just such a circumstance of two people suddenly caught in a negative feedback loop fueled by a stress helicopter looking for a landing pad.

Florence and Edie were chatting while their preteen daughters played around with some costume makeup. The conversation became activating for Florence as she described some intense difficulties her daughter had been facing with *other* friends. Florence tearfully confided in Edie how stressful it had been for Florence's whole family, and how concerned she was feeling, day after day, about her daughter's social connections. Naturally this topic was bringing up some stress reactivity for Florence. What followed indicates that without Florence's knowing it, her stress brain was skewing her sense of today and yesterday. Then her activation helicopter found a place to land, on Edie.

Before that, the preteen girls were happily giggling, listening to music on a smartphone, and applying fun and wild makeup. Suddenly Florence realized she and her daughter were late for an appointment. Hustle and bustle ensued—makeup remover was flying, Edie's daughter was trying to help Florence's as quickly as she could, but it was difficult, and Edie's daughter was working one-handed as she held the music-playing phone in her other hand. The makeup was not coming off easily. Florence, who was already at a 5 or 6 stress level because of her ongoing concern for her daughter's challenging situation—a situation *unrelated* to the here-and-now gathering—was getting more stressed. Her stress level was rising to what appeared to be a 7 or 8.

No one noticed when prescription glasses fell on the floor, and no one meant to step on them—but it happened. No one meant to fill the little cavity of the smartphone with makeup remover, but this too happened. And no one meant to use staining lipstick on anyone's cheeks, eyes, and lips, but they did. The chaos resulted in one makeup-stained face, one broken pair of glasses, and one newly unsmarted phone.

This would be a difficult series of events for anyone, but it sent Florence right into high-stress overload. She was like a well-prepared campfire: once the kindling had been lit, the flames took off. For Florence, her daughter's difficulty with *other* situations was the kindling, and the stress-fueled view of her current situation was the fire. It seemed that Florence could no longer separate her stress of yesterday from her stress of today. She went right into tunnel vision and began to "see" that Edie's daughter had done all of this intentionally. Florence's faulty neuroception led her to believe that Edie's daughter had purposely knocked down the glasses, mishandled the smartphone, and applied the staining makeup all with malicious intent. Florence went so far as to say that Edie's daughter was sabotaging and bullying her intentionally, and that all this chaos was premeditated. Stress brain is good at fabricating ideas like this.

It could have easily been the end of the friendship for these women and their girls. And stress reactivity would have been the unseen culprit. Fortunately, when one nervous system begins to regulate, others systems can often follow suit. Edie had self-regulation in her tool kit and was able to soothe her system. This restored her clear view of the situation. Edie saw the innocence of the girls' play and recognized the unintended chain of mistakes and accidents. Edie's clear seeing and sensing anchored her regulation and enabled her to anchor the whole situation.

As Edie's regulation increased, so did Florence's; she could then see that all the accidents were just that: accidents. After each woman had returned to her own true baseline, both realized there had been no ill will at any point, and that this situation was *not* the same as some in the past.

Everyone recovered from this kerfuffle. But this is real; our brains do this. And when we believe our dysregulated seeing and sensing, things do not always turn out so well. Our faulty neuroception happens all the time. And these misperceptions are elaborate, convincing, *and* a burden; a burden than can be somewhat lightened by tuning in and taking a look around.

TUNING IN TO WHAT IS OKAY

By tuning in to the here and now—particularly to what is okay, pleasant, or pleasurable in the moment—we direct ourselves toward helpful and positive feedback loops. Seeing and sensing in this way can remedy the disposition of our stress brains to scan for what is *not* okay, *un*pleasant, and *un*pleasurable. The habit of negative bias contributes to building and maintaining the negative feedback loops we've been discussing. When stress reactivity has hijacked your mind-body system, skewing your perceptions and sensations, returning to a clear view can be as simple as taking a look around and pausing to feel your own body.

Seeing and sensing is also a way to take a look at the now, to reorient to today if your stress brain has taken you to yesteryear. For those of us with overwhelming stresses in our past, when we return to here and now, we often find *now* is much more manageable than *then*. And seeing and sensing can be a way to take a break—like that moment on an airplane when you fly up out of heavy clouds and fog into a clear blue sky. A seeing break can clear away stress fog and give you a new view of things.

This is powerful stuff. Seeing our environment has a tremendous effect on how we feel, and what we sense has a tremendous effect on what we see. As we learned from Spiderman (and Churchill, Roosevelt, and some French revolutionaries...but I digress), "with great power comes great responsibility." It's a big responsibility because there is speed-dial connectivity between seeing, sensing, *and safety*. If we're unaware, we can scare the wits out of ourselves regularly. Let's wield this influence skillfully. Seeing safety can help us feel safety. Feeling okayness can help us see okayness. Of course, the opposite is also true: feel fear, see fear. One of those options awakens the fear and stress brain, the other doesn't. Which do you choose?

The seeing and sensing skill can be put to task with one of two possibilities: as a helpful, soothing influence or as, well, a much less helpful, less soothing input. As Levine describes, seeing and sensing focuses our attention where the healing can begin. Healing our basic sense of our inner and outer world; healing the mirages of stress brain that some of us live with daily.

BRIEF MOMENTS OF SEEING DO CREATE SHIFTS

There is so much going on around us at any given point, we have to choose to focus on the pertinent information and filter out the rest. However, can we choose to make some of the pleasant and neutral sights around us pertinent? After all, these *are* pertinent to our well-being.

It's not that we need to be constantly scanning and tracking *all* that is around us; a short pause in our directed focus will do. We can briefly shift from tunnel vision, or even an intense but narrow focus, to a more open mode of perception and give our system a substantial nudge toward ease. A brief moment to recognize a lovely shaft of light streaming through a window, or a picture on the wall, or a view of outside, can start a positive feedback loop.

Try It Now

Take a look around. Let your eyes explore your environment. Take your time seeing things around you that may have previously gone unnoticed. Let your eyes choose something, and rest your gaze there for a few moments.

Enjoy. Good for you!

NOTICING THE SUBTLE, TOO

Most of the time, we notice only the big sensations. We tend to tune in to great pleasures like a massage or great aches like a sprained ankle. It's common to miss sensations that are *mildly* pleasant or just okay. When is the last time you really stopped to take in a subtle shift toward relaxation in your jaw, neck, or shoulders, or a release of tightness in your belly, or a relative stillness in your legs, ankles, or feet? Don't know? Those sensations go largely unnoticed by most of us.

Try It Now

Take a moment now to feel any areas of your body that are subtly pleasant or neutral. Scan from your feet up to your head, noticing areas that are quietly okay.

Can you feel your feet on the floor or surface they are touching? Is there a place along your legs where you can feel the chair, couch, ground you are sitting on? Are there areas in your back that are at ease? Can you notice any part of your neck or jaw that feels somewhat comfortable right now? Scan for simple okayness.

Good for you!

Two Peas in a Pod

Using the tool of seeing and sensing sets in motion resilience and well-being. Tuning in to soothing or even just okay sensations and sights can be a game changer—and a brain changer. If you find yourself in persistent negative feedback loops fueled by your perceptions and sensations, the tool of sensing and seeing should become a go-to for you.

HOW TO USE THE TOOL OF SEEING AND SENSING

You can use the tools of seeing and sensing many different ways. Each of us can find our own unique approach. You might use it to find a safe person in the room, as Mary did in the earlier example. You would use a moment of orienting to find a refuge in a stressful environment and undo your negative bias. Sometimes one safe person can direct your entire body-mind system away from Stressville. Or you might direct your seeing and sensing to understanding and seeing the truth of a hectic situation, as was the case with Florence and Edie. When activation is tarnishing yours or others' view and creating false perspectives, seeing and sensing can be part of bringing you back to reality and back to today from yesterday.

We can also use seeing and sensing to interrupt our activation and keep it from overwhelming us, taking a much-needed break from our stress. Helen did this when she put aside the subject of her negative work circumstances for a moment and instead took a look around at her own safe and soothing environment. Seeing and sensing as a refuge from negative bias, an orientating to today, or an interruption of activation are just a few of the many options for this tool. See how it works best for you. Make it yours.

Try This: Easy Seeing and Sensing for Okayness

Try this when you have a little time—when the moment is uncomplicated and things are basically okay. This practice builds a foundation for this tool's other uses. It truly is as simple as taking a look around.

1. Let your eyes scan the area around you. Look near, look far.

2. Allow your eyes to choose something they want to rest on. Ask your eyes what they like looking at.

3. As you look at it, let your gaze just rest there, soft and easy. You may even let your eyes soften to the point of blurring for a moment and then gently bring the object back into focus. The eyes are *receiving* the view you're resting on, not looking out to *get* the view.

4. As you let your eye settle, notice how it feels in your body to be gazing at something pleasant. How does your body respond to this seeing practice you're doing? Scan your body for areas of release or relative ease. Attend to these subtle shifts in your body as you also see your chosen view.

5. Notice how your body feels. Attend to any areas of the body that have eased up a bit or relaxed somewhat with your seeing practice. Take in the sensations of the areas that are okay. Breathe with this awareness for a few moments.

This is not meant to be hard work. This is easy and light. Just invite yourself to see for a few moments. There is no need to do this for long periods of time. Little moments of seeing throughout your day are wonderful for your nervous system. This is resetting you back to baseline. No big effort needed. We can't stress our way *out* of stress. You just bring a little attention, and gently notice what you see and feel.

Easy does it. Less is more.

SEEING DURING STRESS

As we've discussed, in times of stress our brain tunes out the okay things happening around us in favor of focusing on identifying any and all possible threats. So when we are heading toward Stressville, we can take a seeing break. It's like throwing yourself a line while you are adrift in a sea of stress. No need to tune out or try to turn off the stress. This is an "and also" practice. You acknowledge that X stress is occurring, *and also* there is a lovely view out the window from where you sit; or Y stress is right there in front of you, *and also,* you can see your dog curled up sweetly in her bed.

Try This: Seeing During Stress

1. As the stress reactivity begins to take hold, find a moment to take a seeing break.

2. Let your eyes look for something around you that *does not* contribute to the stress. Is there a tree, flower, or ray of sunlight that pleases

your eye? Is there a lovely painting, a pet, or a person nearby that you enjoy seeing?

3. As you take your seeing break, can you feel how it affects your body? Is there anywhere in your body that releases even a degree of tension? Is there any subtle shift toward relief?

4. Let yourself see and feel the okay parts, just for a moment. This will soothe your system a bit and help you go back to the stressor you are facing with some more self-regulation on board.

With these practices, little by little you will build resilience pathways. These pathways will increase neural connectivity between your soothing front brain and your alarmist back brain. Over time, your clear view and soothing sensation awareness will more directly lead to increased regulation. The more you use this tool, the more neural and somatic-resilience pathways you'll build and the stronger and more effective those pathways will be.

CHAPTER 6

A Picture Instead of a Thousand Words

Pictures in the mind pop up all the time for many of us. And they are not always just inconsequential images. For years I had enjoyed hiking the hills near my home, often filled with ease and delight, until one hot summer day when an alarming sight burned itself into my mind—as alarming images are wont to do. While hiking a very familiar trail, all of a sudden, a large snake appeared on the trail in front of me. I screamed. I was scared. It was big. My heart pounded, sweat started to prick at my underarms, and all the muscles in my back squeezed intensely, like I was a nearly empty tube of toothpaste and the muscles along my spine were determined to get the last bit of paste out of me! The snake waggled its head—checking me out, I think. It looked like it might want to defend itself, but then to my great relief, it slithered on.

During the next half-mile or so, still rattled (pun intended) from that unwelcome sighting, my eyes were playing tricks on me. Every stick I passed seemed to be a snake. Really, they were! Except actually, they weren't. But still, every "snake" provoked my heart rate to spike and my knees to buckle all over again. As I continued to hike on, with my fear response activated, my threat scanning was completely on, and I kept "identifying" danger in every shadow, stick, and hole in the ground I passed. And I had the unwanted companions of all the images that flash in your head when you're worried—like a scary preview of what stressful things *might* be up ahead for you. I was swirling with those.

After much self-soothing—rhythmic breathing, orienting to safety whenever I could see it, and sensing any parts of my body that were okay *enough* (a.k.a. using the tools in this book)—I was finally calming down. But you won't believe what happened next. I actually saw another snake, a real one! A big one. My adrenaline shot through my body, again. Think of the high striker at the county fair—the game where you swing a hammer onto the lever, shooting a puck up to ring the bell. My bells were ringing loud and clear throughout my entire body and mind. "Not just one, but two snake meetings," I thought. This fear imprint was now fairly deep in me, and the related mind-body stress reaction from this whole thing did not fade away so quickly.

During the next month of hikes, although my brain knew that the likelihood that I would see another snake was almost nil, my body was not convinced. I would involuntarily brace myself for the possibility of seeing a snake around the next bend on the trail, and whenever I started to unconsciously brace at the possibility, I started to "see" snakes. The sticks really seemed to be slivering around me, I swear! Negative feedback loop. On repeat.

It is not lost on me that in the scheme of things, this is a very mild stressor. For those of you who have faced extreme stressors, amplify this tale, doubling or tripling the intensity; this will give you a pretty good idea of what happens in us humanoids when we're faced with alarming situations. Ask almost anyone if they're familiar with fear-invoking images popping into their mind, uninvited, when they're faced with an anxiety-provoking situation, and most will say yes (and maybe even inundate you with tales of the gruesome things they once imagined). These *imagined* images that just pop up and flash before our eyes can substantially turn up the intensity on the *real* stressor and on our *real* stress reactivity. There is good news in this, however: just as we can scare our whole body-mind system with *negative* imaginings, we can viscerally soothe our body-mind system with *positive* imaginings.

I used positive imagery to work my way back to feeling at ease on those hiking paths again. Not to live in la-la land, but to even things up between the frightening images that were running free in my head. Little by little, I created positive imagery so that paths looked like paths—instead of the negative imagery I had been replaying, which showed paths as snake breeding grounds with loads of slithering beasts waiting to get me! I'm happy to say that with the imagery

This is a flip-the-script approach.

We can *picture* something stressful and feel stressed.

Flip it: We can *picture* something soothing and feel soothed.

work I did concerning my hikes, over time, sticks returned to sticks, and snakes were nowhere to be seen. Using positive imagery to repair negative imagery is what we'll explore in this chapter.

NOT NEW, NOT NEW-AGE

Working with stress images and stressful memories goes back at least a few hundred years. In the late 1800s, Pierre Janet researched stress memories and explained that a stressful event can imprint itself in our minds and bodies and repeat inside us in the forms of images and sensations. Overwhelming memories can be like stressful movies or slide shows that play repeatedly in our minds and then in our bodies.

When this mental movie or slide flashes in our head, it can be a large mental—psychological—event. A cascade of neural reactions takes place as the image plays; thoughts may dance, or an internal dialogue may swirl. But this movie is also a large physical—physiological—event. Heart quickening, sweat starting on the lip or under our arms, knot in the stomach, and headache all can seem to suddenly occur as the stress show begins.

Levine, a master at helping others renegotiate traumatic memories, works with imagery as a central aspect of his therapeutic approach. According to Levine, during extreme-stress events, image memory is heightened and we will often have acute awareness of sights, sounds, and smells. If these stress-related images are not adequately processed, they can be carved into our brain and body. The adrenaline our body secretes during stress events plays a big role in these stress memories becoming engraved in our minds. If we have lived through adrenalized stress experiences that overwhelmed us, or if we have endured stress that we still seem to "feel in our bones," we would be wise to work with the images surrounding those events to sufficiently process the memory and soothe the system.

Beth had successfully battled cancer, yet was finding herself still gripped by fear that it was returning every time some part of her body ached. Each minor pain would lead to a stress-increasing movie dominating her mind. For Beth, a backache became another tumor waiting to be discovered; a headache, a possible brain growth; digestive upset, also cancer. Her rather run-of-the-mill bodily sensations were becoming an on switch to the projector of her mind, launching scary scenes that all ended in her being ill again.

Before Beth and I began working with self-generated positive images, her body was going into full-blown stress reactivity regularly, sometimes multiple times each day. This was debilitating for her and deeply disheartening. Her mind knew that she was doing really well and was several years into her recovery from her initial cancer. She wanted her body to get those facts too. Generating mental movies that *soothed instead of scared her system* was a game changer for her. With each new soothing movie and slide she created, the stress reaction cycle weakened and the stress-resilience cycle strengthened. Again, we are not rewriting history; we are rewiring physiology. The image is a prompt for your body to go toward resilience instead of stress.

Long-Lasting Internal Movies

Even after substantial time has passed, stress memories can be reactivated by images and sounds around us and within us. This is where flashbacks come from. Think of a car backfiring and causing a war veteran to drop onto his belly on the sidewalk and cover his head—a sound triggers all kinds of internal images and sensations. My own daughter, having suffered from a bad accident that took place in a doorway, felt a rush of fear whenever she saw doorjambs or people standing in doorways for more than a year after her accident. She would involuntarily tremble, feel panicked, and flash back to her accident just at the sight of a setting similar to that of her accident.

Jennifer had been working in a very stressful work environment for just over a year. Her company started each new employee with a probationary period and then closely watched all staff to ensure that work policies were upheld. Under these pressures, Jennifer was suffering from system-wide stress reactivity. Intrusive images of her stressful work environment would involuntarily pop up when she wasn't at work and regularly trigger full-bodied stress and dis-ease.

> If an image is similar to one of our unresolved stress imprints, our body and mind can easily get confused. In this confusion, our primitive brain will treat the *similar image* as the *real thing* and go into full-fledged reactivity.

When we are overwhelmed by stress images, our modern brain shuts down and we are left dependent on the nonverbal primitive lobes that govern emotion and sensation. These emotion and sensation centers include the amygdala, seated deep within the fear-driven parts of the brain, and the brain stem, where a great deal of our automatic physical responses are administered.

In this emotion and sensation part of the brain, a switch can flip, causing a racing heart, a spike or sudden drop in body temperature, dry mouth, knot in the stomach, or chest tightness. All this can stem from the cascade of uninvited images in our heads that were spawned by that reminder we just saw or heard—like a doorway for my daughter or a car backfire for a war veteran. The skills in this chapter will help reduce or alter these unwanted movies and slides. The film crew here will use everything available: thoughts, sensations, emotions, and of course, those pictures in the mind.

Try This: Exploring Internal Movies or Slides

Let's get acquainted with some internal movies or slides

You may already know the powerful influence your internal images can have on your whole body-mind system. For many, this will be brand new. Let's play with it a bit.

1. Choose a *positive* memory that is vivid enough for you to be able see the place you were in, the people with you, and what was happening there. Let yourself take a few moments to picture the whole scene. Spend some time inside this memory, recalling any details you can. No need to be historically precise; you can embellish or take your best guess. Just make sure you stay in the positive details of the memory.

2. Now notice how hanging out in this memory feels in your body *right now*. You are not trying to remember how you felt in your body then. Right here, right now, what happens in your chest, belly, shoulders, neck, face, and so on when you conjure this memory and revel in it a little?

3. Now let's explore a *somewhat negative* memory. Again, picture the place, the players, the circumstances. Spend some time in it; see, hear, even smell what was happening there.

4. Now again notice what happens in your body *right now*. What do your belly, chest, neck, back, and so on feel like in this moment? Is it different from what happened in your body during the positive image?

5. Don't stay here long. Take a look around and see something in your environment that you enjoy. Take a few slow and low breaths. Come back to today.

6. If you still feel like part of you is in the negative memory, take time to listen to some of your favorite music, have a cup of tea, take a short walk, or call a friend.

7. Come back to today, to what is okay here and now.

Good for you!

I hope your body showed you how linked internal images and physical sensations are. Current research affirms this too.

Images Affect Your Body and Mind, and They Are Changeable

In decades of research, from 1975 through 2005, psychologist Elizabeth Loftus demonstrated the malleability of memory. Perhaps her most famous body of research is a series of studies coined as "lost in a mall" studies (Loftus and Pickrell 1995; Loftus 2005). Participants in several of these studies were told about four memories from their childhood. Three of the memories were actually true and accurate historical accounts collected from family members, while the fourth "memory" was made up by the scientists and involved being lost in a mall as a young child. The circumstances of where the participants were lost and who finally found them were described to the study participants in detail. Later, when participants were asked to "remember" their experience of getting lost in a mall, many of them believed they had actually been lost. Some participants described visual details; some said they remembered feeling afraid. Interestingly, some of the made-up mall memories actually became stronger over time; the participants felt even more drawn in by these implanted "memories" weeks after the mall story had first been told to them.

In another study, Björkstrand and colleagues (2015) determined that *renegotiating* negative memories during recall significantly lowers the stress reactivity for that memory. These scientists measured amygdala reactivity and sweat production with memory renegotiation. The results showed that when negative images were *interrupted and reformed* right after recall, the person's amygdala activity and sweat production decreased. In an eighteen-month follow up, these results persisted. The study participants, who had interrupted their negative memories eighteen months before, continued to have less fear-brain reactivity and sweating related to that memory. The results also showed that interrupting fearful and stressful memories would require less mental effort, especially in the fear brain. This will free up precious brainpower for connecting with friends and family, focusing on work, and even just remembering where your keys are.

> If an image was implanted in a person's memory, their mind-body system took it to be real, whether it actually happened or was imagined.

Collectively, these studies indicate that the mental movie does not have to be true, nor something we've actually lived, in order to bring about strong mental, emotional, and physical reactions. We can have just as robust a reaction to a self-created "memory" as a real one. This can put us in the driver's seat of our brain-body system, wherein we support ourselves in creating images, movies, and slides that soothe instead of stress.

EVOLUTIONARY THEORY

"Why does my brain and body do this?" It seems that the humans who survived eons ago were really good at *mentally recording dangerous images* in their minds and having that information at the ready so that they could consult it at a moment's notice—essentially memorizing the top hits that would come up in a Google query of "what is dangerous or threatening to me."

If we were living outside on the plains, and our daily task was to just stay alive, we would need to be *very clear* about what did and did not pose a threat to us. If we saw a small bird flying toward us, for example, we would need to know *This one is safe; do not freak out.* If instead we saw a lion running toward us, we would need to know quickly *This one is not safe; proceed to freak out.* In primitive times, humans couldn't quickly consult Wikipedia on a smartphone when they saw the shape of an elephant in the distance for a quick confirmation of what that looming shape was. Nor did they have the luxury of closing and locking all doors and windows while establishing just how threatening any given situation might be.

Flash forward to now. When our brain-body system identifies something as a threat, even a small one, we are very likely to mine this thousands-of-years-old skill and begin looping said dangerous scenario in our minds. Both real and imagined slides and movies will play in the background of our mind, while our stress and fear physiology ramps up and up and up. As our jaw clenches, stomach tightens, and limbs tremble, our body is gearing up to defend itself or run away. All while we are actually just sitting there remembering stressful events that have passed or imagining possible stress events yet to come.

> The primitive brains of our ancestors seem to have evolved with an uncanny ability to create slideshows and self-made documentaries starring the most fearful and dangerous aspects of their lives and had them in the background of their minds on an endless loop as they went about their other cave-related errands.

THE BODY DOESN'T DIFFERENTIATE WELL

What's more, when we feel extreme stress, our bodies are in a reaction very similar to that of our ancestors' bodies. *They* might have been facing tigers. *We* might be facing public speaking. But our bodies do not know the difference. To the body, extreme stress is extreme stress, and extreme stress wakes up the survival brain and calls in the troops from the nervous system.

Alexandra related to me that when she stood in front of an audience of people to give a talk, it felt like a group of alligators were sitting before her, ready to eat her up! Flashes of negative images would take over her mind, making it hard for her to breathe or simply stand up, let alone think and speak—her mind became flooded with terrifying images and her body reacted by nearly fainting.

THE INTERNAL SHOW CAN START ALL TOO EASILY

For people with extreme-stress imprints, difficult images are common. Various circumstances are likely to prompt stress images to replay, and large or small triggers stimulate the stress slideshow to begin.

Over the years, Cynthia had unfortunately faced several serious situations that threatened the well-being of her children. She was no stranger to the emergency room and had been through more than her fair share of very serious circumstances.

It's not unusual for overwhelm to occur in situations that might seem manageable to people who do not have a history of extreme stress and do not suffer from intrusive images. Remember, it is not your current circumstance that's causing your reactivity, but your historic imprint that is giving rise to your body-mind eruptions.

> Pierre Janet emphasized that if we are *overwhelmed* by stress during our stressful events, our memories don't process sufficiently. Unprocessed memories lead to fearsome intrusive images.

Cynthia was becoming increasingly worried about her children's progress at school; her children's well-being often acted as a trigger for her. When she saw her children falling behind in school, their marks dropping, her stress levels rose significantly. Uninvited mental images first had her seeing her kids failing the year-end exams. Then not getting accepted to the secondary school they had applied for. This progressed to seeing them not attending college. And her final image was of her adult children living out their days in her basement. Cynthia shared this with a bit of humor, yet while she tried to be lighthearted about this far-fetched chain of images, she was also feeling the real effects of stress throughout her body-mind. Her intrusive stress images were magnifying her reactivity, keeping her up at night, contributing to migraines, and inducing panic.

While these kinds of invasive images are very common for us extreme-stress sufferers, they're still very painful, and even debilitating. The next exercise can help you inventory what triggers these for you.

Explore This

What Are Your Common Stress Cues or Triggers?	
People • People who have mistreated you or your loved ones • Loved ones who have been threatened or in danger • People in positions of power or authority • People in great need or dependency	Places • Places you've been hurt or scared • Places you've felt incapacitated or diminished • Places you've felt trapped or stranded • Places you've been singled out or persecuted
Sounds • Certain noises • Certain voices • Too much or too little sound	Scents • Smells that remind you of negative situations • Smells of a certain place, person, or time
Kinds of emotions or thoughts • Worry • Fear • Anger • Sadness • Violence	Sensations • Temperature (hot/cold) • Shakiness • Tension • Dizziness • Numbness • Confinement
Situations • Dangerous • Rushed • Pressured • Trapped • Lonely • Helpless	Things • Objects • Colors • Textures

Van der Kolk describes triggers as traces of the original event. When these traces rekindle sensations of *historic* stress events, the *original* stress response is reignited in the body. We can be standing in front of a building that any passerby can see is in perfectly fine condition, but our body can be reacting as if the whole thing is on fire. Fortunately for us, the reverse is also true. Situations and images that we associate with safety, ease, and protection can also ignite reliable responses in the body. We can take time, in a safe space, to process that house on fire and slowly return our system to balance at the sight of similar buildings.

Richard was working one summer as a house painter and fell off of a two-story building. He was alone when it happened. He sought my help because many years later, whenever he saw ladders, high-rise construction, and other settings that presented a similar risk of falling, he would vividly reexperience the tremors of pain and the terror of being alone and injured. He wanted to feel differently about these sights, to feel less pulled into his bodily reactivity when he thought of that summer so long ago. He was aware that over time, parts of his memory had amplified the event and it had become progressively worse.

Research shows that when we pull a memory or mental image into our minds, it is in a somewhat neurally translucent state, meaning the image is not entirely solid yet, not a fully formed memory. In this translucent state, we can either confirm the old memory or alter it. When we confirm a memory as it was before, we elicit the same physical reaction that we initially had. The same fear-inducing image produces the same headache, sweating, jaw tension, and so on that we experienced the first time our minds made that movie. And often, the sweating and headache of today *increase* our alarm, and the original image *worsens* each time we pull the memory up. We've probably all known someone whose first successfully caught fish gets several inches longer, bigger, and more difficult to reel in each time they retell the tale. Their body is cueing them to *intensify* the story; the adrenaline coursing through them is causing the embellishment, not just the fun of a great story.

If we take advantage of this neural translucence and create an image that *deescalates* our reactivity, this old image won't be able to sink its claws into us as it once did. A new image that induces calm instead of stress means a milder headache or none at all, less sweating, a relaxed jaw, and so on.

Richard played with a few different options within his memory. He imagined slowing down the fall a great deal, instead of the speed that played a major role in his overwhelm. As he pictured himself falling very slowly, his body began to do something very different. A relaxing in his back, belly, and throat replaced the intense constriction that was usually there when he recalled that day. His terror softened into an alertness that was much more manageable for him, and with this, his heart rate slowed considerably, which lessened his overall fear reactivity. He then decided to imagine that someone *had* been there when he hit the ground, instead of the terrible aloneness he had experienced. He chose a good friend whom he knew would have been supportive and caring and imagined this good friend next to him as he lay on the ground, stunned. With this imagined support, Richard teared up a little, and he felt the long-held isolation that accompanied this memory begin to recede. Richard basked in this image for a moment and felt the release that would have been possible had it all taken place more slowly and with friendly support available to him at the time. The good news was, it was available to him now, and his reaction to the memory was dramatically changed as a result of his reconfiguring the image a little.

We are not rewriting history—not at all. We are flipping the script on the negative movies and slide shows that we *unintentionally* play in our minds when stress comes knocking. We are *intentionally* playing some "clips" of positive images. We are counterbalancing the weight of the damaging memories.

Remember, thanks to evolution, our primitive minds and bodies are hell-bent on memorizing possible danger. So it's up to the modern brain-body to balance out those mental pictures. When we counterbalance, and even out the scales, our system is soothed. When our system is soothed, we feel good, think clearly, and have access to "nonessentials" like creativity, empathy, light-heartedness, and knowing what's happening now and what's history. This is self-regulation via imagery.

Try This: Self-Regulation via Imagery

1. Think of a stressor that happened too unexpectedly or without the support of others.

2. Give yourself a moment to picture where you were, what happened, how it unfolded.

3. Notice what happens in your body as you remember this scenario. What do your chest, belly, back, throat, legs, and arms feel like?

4. Now experiment with reconfiguring this image a little. What if you slow it all down? What if you added the presence of a trusted friend, or someone you deeply respect? If that trusted person had been there, what might they have said or done?

5. Give yourself time to picture these new additions to this memory. You might notice you feel differently as this goes along.

6. This might not be the right alteration for you within this memory. If so, see if you'd like to try a different version of the vision. Experiment until you find one that works.

Remember: We're not changing the truth; we're soothing the way our body reacts to the truth. You're still going to know what *did* happen, the next time you think about that memory. But your heart may not beat as fast, and you may not feel sweat beads forming on your lip after you've shared a soothing mental image of more okayness with your nervous system.

Maria created a simple image reconfiguration that she played with during a stress-filled and dysregulated period of her life. She reimagined the faces of the people she was about to interact with. Having grown up in an often-hostile environment and then years later found herself working in an often-hostile environment, fear of a harsh reception kept surfacing for her. Maria didn't *want* to picture the anticipated reception as one of rejection, but it kept popping up just as she was heading out the door for somewhere new. Images of unfriendliness would flash through her mind and the accompanying bodily tremors would follow.

So Maria began to flip it. She would take some time to imagine a few welcoming, kind, or warm faces somewhere in the group she was about to encounter. Then she'd take time to *feel* what this image did in her body; her throat would soften, heart rate slow, and stomach unclench. Because of these brief moments of image reconfiguration, as she walked into these unfamiliar situations, she was more or less regulated and had access to much more of her creative and connecting front brain.

This is one way we can even the scales of negative to positive images in the mind. When we are in a pattern of making up negative "what-ifs," we would be wise to *make up* some positive possibilities as well. When we are projecting future possibilities, the negative images are just that: possibilities. Yet our body-mind system is taking them as a certain or likely future—and these so-called predictions are freaking us out.

> We are not rewriting history, we are rewiring physiology.

IT CAN START IN THE MIND OR IN THE BODY

Stressful images can prompt stress sensations, and stress sensations can prompt stressful images. If your system has been living in a state of high stress, the cycle loops.

Body-to-mind stress can happen all too easily. Remember my snake encounter? Skip forward to many months later: I'm hiking and listening to a podcast; it isn't even snake season any longer. This podcast I'm listening to is covering a really hard-to-hear but important subject, and my fear response is becoming activated by what I'm hearing. I feel my tension rising, my emotions transitioning from okay to fearful. And then suddenly, I watch my brain switch into a now long-past mode. The sticks begin to look like snakes again. My body response to the podcast—shallow breathing, spike in heart rate, excessive tension in my gut, and so on—cues my mind that something must be wrong, and in comes the mind to crack the case, and then see snakes. A.k.a. self-generate fear-related imagery.

We can all feel stressed and then unwittingly *picture* stressful images in our mind. This cycle has to do with how deeply connected our body and mind are, and how singularly focused our whole system can become when we experience high levels of activation. When we feel intensely stressed, our stress-driven brain switches into danger-scanning mode, in which the brain often perceives *only* evidence that supports its point of view. We miss entire aspects of reality in this stress-driven brain. Remember that evolution has survival as our first order of business. When we're tracking the *threat*—a lion, for example—we are not noticing the beautiful sunset behind the giant figure of the fierce beast. Who has extra brain space to bother with a lovely pink hue at a time like this!

According to Robert Sapolsky, when the stress is primarily psychological, as is the case with mental images and narratives, the distress our system unleashes can actually be more detrimental to us than the actual stressor itself. After all, with psychological stress, what is *actually* taking place is only a mental image or internal narrative playing in the mind, but what is happening in the body can be a large, uncomfortable or even painful stress response! During my hike with the snakes and sticks, it wasn't that mistaking sticks for snakes was such a huge problem for the few months it persisted. The problem was that my body-mind system kept scaring itself. The bigger issue was that with each fright I endured, the fear response was becoming ever more deeply engrained in my system. Many of us suffer from this predicament: our stress response is so deeply engrained that it pops up whether we really need it or not. In these instances, we can rely on soothing our feelings of stress with images that engender ease.

Professionally and personally, I've seen that during intensely stressful periods, even moderately stressful events can evoke stress images, movies, or slides. When our mind-body system is out of balance, tipping toward stress overload, the body and brain stress reaction is at the ready. With our stress reaction on such a hair trigger, negative images are often close to the surface of the mind and become a regular part of how our body-mind does stress.

HOW TO USE THE TOOL OF REGULATING IMAGERY

With this tool, we can counterbalance the compelling power of the fear-driven primitive brain with positive imagery from our modern brain and even out the scales of the two.

Step one: Learn to recognize your body's stress reaction: heart rate increase, dry mouth, tense neck or shoulders, stomachache, trembling, going numb, etc. Keep in mind that each of us has our own stress signature, our body's unique response to high pressure or overwhelm.

Step two: Become aware of the images, movies, or slides that pop up in your mind during your stress reactions. Being able to recognize when stress—and not the what-ifs—is the real lead actor in your mental show will be very helpful for changing how the scene ends.

Step three: Ask yourself, "If this could have gone differently, what would have been less stressful for me?" Let your mind wander a bit; sometimes the answer is very realistic, sometimes it's really based in fantasy. Either, or both, can have a tremendously positive effect on your nervous system.

Step four: Consult a menu of options for imagery reconfiguration; more simply put, your imagined do-over.

Your Movie Menu

Somatic therapy has shown that there are a few dependable approaches to self-regulating imagery. I like to think of it as a short menu from which to choose. Let me give you an example. After a tight election race, when my preferred candidate didn't win, I had a fitful night of sleep, wracked with nightmares of what might be yet to come. I woke up with a start, simultaneously hot and cold, heart pounding, neck and shoulders clenched tight, with images from my dreams flooding my head. As I lay there in the dark, I said to myself, *Rebekkah, you are terrifying yourself.* The pictures flashing through my mind were terrible. I began to go through my image menu and *ask my body* which item it liked best. Remember: this is not a brain decision; this is a body decision. The item I chose was the one that helped slow my heart and relax my shoulders and neck and returned me to the knowledge

> Your felt experience is your guide. These are body decisions, not brain choices.

that at that exact moment, at 2 a.m., in my quiet house, things were okay.

When your stress reaction is activated and spiraling out of control like this, you can consult a menu of possibilities, just as I did to relieve my activation and reach a state of okayness.

Menu:

Item 1: A Support

Item 2: A Boundary

Item 3: A Defense

Item 4: A Resolution

Item 5: A Time Adjustment

As you consult your menu, your body sensations are paramount. This is not a mental choice or an evolved brain choice; this is gut level. Let your body choose an image that really *feels* relieving. What does it *feel* like to imagine a less-stressful outcome? Does imagining a support do the trick? Does the presence of a boundary help more? Would having things slow down lead you to *feel* that you can finally curl up in the evolutionary grass to rest and recover? Who knows? Maybe you'll bump into some nice zebras there.

Item 1: A Support

As mentioned in chapter 2, before our system goes into flight, fight or freeze/shutdown mode, there is first an instinct to seek support. An ally, a protector, or a trusted companion can make all the difference to our stress brain. Sometimes the aloneness of our stress is central to the overwhelm we feel. We can add a support by picturing someone there at the scene with us. Maybe someone we know—it could even be someone we've never met. Archetypal figures can be very supportive as well as strangers we admire. Animals can be deeply relieving to our system too. Sometimes there is just a quick moment of picturing a good friend, one you know has your back, standing with you as you faced that difficult situation.

You can also imagine that someone who *was* there, picturing them as having been more available and consoling to you then they actually were. Maybe the person you were with was also lost in their stress brain and the two of you spiraled together. Imagining that person being more present, kind, or emotionally responsive can be a huge change for your body-mind system.

Item 2: A Boundary

This can be as simple as imagining something between you and the negative situation, person, or place. A wall? A forest? A shield? An ocean? Sometimes people feel safer if they picture having been just a few streets away, or a few buildings down the street. Sometimes picturing wrapping yourself up in a cozy blanket becomes the protective boundary that would have benefited you during that stressful time. If you could have had anything between you and that ugly scene, what might it be? Let yourself see that, and notice how it *feels*.

Item 3: A Defense

This menu item can feel taboo, and it's not the best choice for every situation, but for some, it fits like a glove. I joke with my clients, "No one will be harmed in the making of this image." This is a moment to let the primitive—your reactive and certainly not polite—brain have its way. When we give our primitive brain a few minutes to picture self-protection—a fair impulse, if you ask me—we can then actually move on from repeatedly *enacting* self-protection. Ever get caught in defensiveness when you're upset? I know I have been. Sometimes letting your *mental* movie defend you keeps you from bullheadedly going at the person *actually* standing across from you.

Item 4: A Resolution

Sometimes, our fear brain has us fixate on the bad part of a stress event and we hardly see or feel how it all worked out. Seeing and feeling that final resolution can remind your system that it can lay that old burden down, and with it, all the unnecessary activation that this historic stress event is still causing. And if there might have been a better conclusion to that stress event than what actually occurred, you can picture that too. Sometimes people picture it as a yet-to-have-taken-place conclusion. Seeing that in the future, things will feel much more resolved than they do now. And you'll feel how much ease those reassurances bring to body and mind.

Item 5: A Time Adjustment

Often, slowing things down can make a huge difference in how our nervous system responds to the stress event. Adjusting the time frame of a stress memory can give you time to prepare for the yucky thing that is up ahead in that memory. In contrast, sometimes speeding through certain sections feels much better than lingering. However you decide to use this time-shifting, time can be on your side in a way that it might not have been if you didn't take time to rework a stress image.

Further Inspiration for Using the Menu Items

In his 2004 book *Why Zebras Don't Get Ulcers,* Sapolsky explains, well, just that. Zebras, being the clever mammals that they are, have instincts, and they follow them. They follow those instincts until the drive is gone—and hopefully the threat is gone too—and then circle up together in the grass to rest and recover. We, on the other hand, can try to squash our instincts and get on with trying to pass ourselves off as unaffected humans.

If your primitive brain does not get time to follow through with its impulses, either in reality or through an image, it keeps readying itself for the moment when it will finally be able to protect you. This could have an evolutionary basis too; if there was a tiger pacing near your cave opening but not coming in, you didn't forget about it and go back to watching cave-flix. You stayed keyed up, ready to react as soon as the threat got any more serious. Those cave dwellers, who had registered that there was some danger lurking and had not yet reacted to that stressor, had a survival system telling them to stay geared up in case they need to quickly react to the threat later. In our modern world, later never comes, and we bury our self-protection instincts deep within our bodily tissues. They hide there, but they don't rest. They become ulcers, migraines, insomnia, irritable bowels, chronic infection, panic attacks, persistent anxiety, and all the rest of it.

Zebras don't suffer from lasting *mental* stress, either. A huge reason they don't get ulcers is that they don't replay their stresses in their heads. Awake at night worrying about home-equity line of credit? Not the whales. Fretting over a fight with an ex-husband? Not the kangaroo. Lost in anger about a recent insult from another herd? Not the rhinos. Since we humans have uniquely busy minds, and we do not seem to be able to just stop all those internal images from flashing upstairs, let's use some of that mental muscle to our advantage and have some creative do-overs in our heads. When the event is actually long over but still living on inside your gut, or when your stress response is significantly greater than the actual stressor, or when the what-if scenario that ends in catastrophe is actually the greatest threat to your health, then image reconfiguration can be just what the doctor ordered.

At-a-Glance Guide to Self-Regulation Through Imagery

1. Recall a time when you had a noticeable stress reaction, or picture a future what-if that has been nagging at you. Picture the time, place, and circumstances.

2. See the mental movie of how it went, or how you think it might go.

3. Notice how this feels in your body:
   - Tight?
   - Hot?
   - Shaky?
   - Stiff?
   - Something else?

4. Check in with your gut, your heart, your throat.

5. Now flip the script. If it could have gone differently, what would have been less stressful?

    •   A Support: A good friend or person you admire was by your side.

    •   A Boundary: You were safely shielded behind something tall or strong.

    •   A Defense: You were able to protect yourself, fight back.

    •   A Resolution: You skip to the end and see how it all plays out, how it resolves.

    •   A Time Adjustment: Slow things down or speed certain parts up.

6. Now *feel* what happens next in your body. How is your gut, heart, or throat?

7. Keep playing with your image until you get some relief; even just a little shift to relief is great. We don't need big huge shifts. Little shifts are like a stepping-stone placed on your new resilience pathway.

Examples of Each Menu Item

With my own example of awakening from nightmares feeling gripped with fear, I went through my menu, and my body liked a wall of protectors best (#1 support and #2 boundary). I imagined a whole team of protectors who work in government to be watchdogs for all citizens. I felt a slight release in my chest with this image, then let myself bask in it as my breathing began to deepen and my muscles began to unclench. Little by little, my body felt *safe enough*. It wasn't that I felt or had imagined that the whole world was perfect and I had just won a trip to the Bahamas. No. I was just prompting my body toward its resilience, finding a do-over of some of my nightmare images. Then I could curl up, not in the grass, but in my bed, and get back to sleep.

My client with young children doing some academic catch-up felt soothed by an image of a resolution (#4 from the menu) and time adjustment (#5). She let herself "see" her kids learning their math facts little by little and improving their reading comprehension slowly but surely.

She imagined into the future and saw that they would eventually get it, and would not be living out their days in her basement after all.

Richard felt great relief from slowing his fall from the second story down (#5). This additional time helped him prepare for the fall within his somatic memory and changed the way he felt about his eventual moment of impact with the ground.

Beth, who successfully fought cancer, at times imagined a wise elder relaying to her that her cancer had passed, a support (#1). At other times, she focused on the good news her oncologist had shared about her being cancer free in her test results, a resolution (#4), and she imagined this into the future.

Another client I worked with pictured a beautiful garden between her and some very stressful people in her life, a boundary (#2). Still another found relief in letting herself imagine fighting back (a defense) after being really mistreated by some members of her family years ago (#3). This client told me she wanted to preserve her relationship with her family but wanted to get the anger and stress out of her body. I explained that within the safety of our sessions was the perfect place to let her primitive brain defend itself so that she could get it out of her system while still having the current civil relationship she had worked so hard to cultivate.

Using the power of images in the mind to our advantage can serve us well. I encourage you to give yourself plenty of time to get the hang of this skill. Practice with small stressors, then work your way up to medium-sized stress events. If you have a large stress event that you'd like to work with, I encourage you to consult a somatic therapist to support you in that process. Be patient with your brain and body; it may currently have a very robust stress response and a rather weak resilience pathway. Little by little, one image at a time, you can rebuild your resilience pathway and guide your body-mind system onto that pathway as needed. Add this skill to your mind-body tool kit, and have it available to you when it fits the situation.

CHAPTER 7

Moving into Your Body

I hope by now you're *inspired* about your body and *excited* by your body, and that you are *in* your body. Yet truly, it's not at all uncommon to *have* a body and nonetheless not be *in* it very much of the time. (James Joyce famously wrote, "Mr. Duffy lived a short distance from his body.") This chapter will offer ways to move into your body by moving your body. To *reinhabit* your body or to *continue to inhabit* your body, movement can be a powerful aid. An aid that brings you back to yourself, back *into* yourself. This is an aid we all need—being *in* ourselves; as they say at every raffle drawing, "You must be present to win." The winnings in this case are a regulated body that feels soothed, secure, and steady, and a regulated mind that can be creative, connecting, and clear. A soothed body and clear mind frees you up from survival mode. When you are no longer burdened with constantly saving your life, you can really start living your life. Getting moving helps you in getting this prize!

This chapter offers three different approaches to movement. First, movement as a source of self-regulation. This is like the sensing practice from chapter 5, only in motion: walking and taking in the comforting sensations of the moment; cycling and feeling the release from the action and coordination of your legs; dancing or stretching with awareness of your body and enjoying the way gravity moves through you.

> Move for:
>
> A body that is *soothed, secure,* and *steady*
>
> A mind that is *creative, connecting,* and *clear*

With the second approach, we'll cover movement as another method of vagal nerve toning. There are simple, easy movements that wake up and tone the vagus, and that complement the breathing practices I described in chapter 4 to help engage your vagus.

Finally, we'll cover how movement can become a powerful tool to help thaw the ice of the freeze response and help us get back to our embodied and ambulant selves. This will include subtle movements that help to start that thawing, as well as full-bodied movements that can help to break long-held patterns of immobility.

MOVING AS A SOURCE OF SOOTHING

Movement can be like chicken soup for the soul; something warm that goes down nice and easy. In service of somatic regulation, we each need to find our own way to move and our own circumstances to move in: Slow or fast? Short or long? Outside or inside? Alone, with a few, or with many? It's all up to your body, what you need, what helps you unfurl into yourself, and what helps you feel the experience of *being in* the body you *live in*. Let us not forget that this body, the one you're in right now, is your first and last home. And the place you'll live throughout your life.

When using movement as a source of self-regulation, it's essential to find the movement that truly does go down nice and easy for you. Your enjoyment is your best guide. No need to push, or strain, or excel. You just need to find a way to move that your muscles and bones, your skin and your breath, the whole of you takes pleasure in.

I was visiting my chiropractor when he said, "Have you heard, sitting is said to be the new smoking?" Well, that's motivation, I thought. That being said, let's not be extremist about this—I've tried that and seen that, and it doesn't help. Movement extremism led me right into several injuries, and I've seen it invoke a neuroticism about exercise that then had to be undone. So...let's not move like that. Maybe sitting isn't exactly the new smoking. But let's make time for this important privilege we've been given, anyway. The important privilege? Having a body. A body that gets to spend some time moving. And of course some time sitting too.

Move to Soothe Your Brain

Tears of relief ran down Samantha's cheeks as she cycled her heart out during her weekly class. These cycle sessions had become a ritual for her during a very stressful time in her life.

Molly danced in a group that met for something that could be described as a movement meditation. The dancers were encouraged to move with and through whatever they might be carrying with them that day. Molly used the dance to move beyond the emotional weight she was accustomed to carrying, each gesticulation helping her to become free of those burdens.

Jeff whooped with pure joy as he biked along a secluded path in a nature preserve near his home, feeling elated as his breath, muscles, and focus all met with the task of riding the mountain.

For Beverly, the freedom of walking out the door and away from the stresses inside her house was a huge relief that trickled down her back and spread to her lower belly. The reassurance of the wide-open sky and space all around her was palpable. She let herself cry and sigh and instinctively move through the tensions that had been building inside her.

Ian used to joke that he was like a dog, as he had to take himself out for walks often or he didn't function very well.

For the extremely stressed, these are not just forms of exercise or simple body maintenance; these are wellness practices. In service of these wellness practices, the key is the *awareness of the release* that the movement facilitates. With the addition of awareness, the soothing benefit of the movement can imprint onto the nervous system and create a positive feedback loop. The embodied consciousness of your relief, or joy, or ease helps to set that somatic experience into your cells. As the neuropsychologist and author Rick Hansen teaches, we do well for ourselves when we take a moment to take in the good. Taking in the goodness that our body feels with movement aids us in absorbing those positive experiences instead of letting the moment slip by without much notice—or much of a lasting imprint.

Feeling the good of movement brings the simple act of moving to a whole new level. In the absence of bodily awareness, the physical tissues of your body will still absorb the benefits of movement: the locomotive muscles will strengthen, the heart and lungs will too. However, when you add the awareness of your body's ease *and* take in that good, or become aware of what feels okay in your body as a result of the movement *and* take that in for a moment, your primitive brain is then invited to the party.

Body awareness is especially effective communication for your primitive brain, because *sensation* is the primitive brain's *native language*.

Let Yourself Take It In

Noticing and taking in what is okay in your body as you move is the practice that soothes your brain—a regulated brain, that is. For a dysregulated brain, you can attend to all the places that are most certainly *not* okay and very successfully spin yourself out. Just as with the seeing practice from chapter 5, where we practiced seeing okayness and *taking in* that we were seeing something okay, with this section's practice, we are moving with some degree of okayness *and taking it in*; feeling where there may be a release of tension or a development of pleasure stemming from the movement, *and taking in* these releases and pleasures, instead of stepping over these moments. When we allow ourselves to take in our releases, take in our pleasures, and take in our well-being, these releases and pleasures become *lived experiences*. These lived experiences facilitate the very well-being we are looking for.

> Awareness of pleasant sensations helps promote positive feedback loops and lets you feel your nervous system's self-regulating power.

As with all somatic practices, easy does it. No need to work hard to take in the ease. Burrowing your awareness into *really* feeling the pleasure of the moment is not what is called for here (yes, I speak from personal experience). This is a light touch of presence, a momentary awareness of okayness, or gently attending to your sensations as a physical release travels through you.

Try This: Moving to Soothe

The next time you're walking, cycling, dancing, stretching, swimming, or engaging in other movement, can you take a moment to feel its positive effects on you? Small or simple experiences of feeling a "yes" anywhere in your body are all that's required. Perhaps there is a little lightness in your disposition, a relief in your chest, a lifting of tension, a pleasure in a deep breath?

It doesn't have to be much. Just a moment of noticing if there is any positive impact of movement. Less is more. And less is plenty.

An easy awareness gives your body a little fuel for regulation. No big deal; just be you sensing your body. Good for you!

The Science of Taking It In

In a study with 147 physical education teachers, all female and middle-aged, the effects of four different kinds of physical activity were examined. The study shed light on how awareness impacted the benefits of movement. Yoga, Feldenkrais, swimming classes, and aerobics were compared to one another, and a computer class was used as a control group. The results showed that the yoga, Feldenkrais, and swimming classes significantly lowered participants' anxiety levels and increased their well-being, whereas the aerobics and computer classes did not. The study correlated this difference with the body awareness and presence that is engendered in the yoga, Feldenkrais, and swimming classes. The scientists concluded that mindful awareness of movement produces positive mood changes (Netz and Lidor 2003).

FIELD NOTES FROM AN MBR STUDY

On a rainy afternoon, the women in my MBR study entered our classroom in various states of stress. One had come from a negative meeting with her child's learning aides, legally required for her child's unique developmental circumstances; another was grappling with the tragic death of a young father in her community; a mother of young children was facing her own recovery from a recent life-threatening diagnosis; and others were facing financial challenges and marital strife, as well as long-held anxieties and tensions.

We stood in a circle gently moving and breathing. Some of us felt our hair damp along our necks as we tilted our heads from side to side, still wet from the dash from car to classroom. Some of us standing in rain boots, most of us in jeans, all of us still a little chilled. Yet with each movement, each awareness of our own ease or our own okayness, the shifts happened. After a few brief stretches, I began to feel my own shoulders soften and looked out at the group to see theirs were too. While stretching our torsos from side to side and being encouraged to feel what was okay in our bodies, I could see a lightening of everyone's mood taking place and feel my own mood shifting right along with them. After less than ten minutes, we sat and checked in. From these few moments of moving and breathing, the group members reported feeling a bit better, a little calmer, and generally more at ease. I could see it in their soft but present eyes, recognize it in their relaxed breathing, hear it in their tone of voice—all of which are impacted by the vagus. And I could feel that all of us had been able to, in just a few moments, help ourselves arrive and settle. Movement can be that powerful.

Moving with awareness and with some attention to the okayness within your body is a very valuable tool for many who seek more self-regulation. Experiment with your movement; find what, where, and how it soothes you. Your enjoyment can be your guide. If you listen in, your body will usually tell you what it likes best.

Next we'll explore the second approach to inhabiting your regulated body by taking a trip to your vagus.

MOVING TO YOUR VAGUS

Moving to Vegas, with all the lights and activity? No. Moving your body in a way that tones your vagus—your important braking system that slows, soothes, and reminds your body-mind of its access to safety. The long "wandering" nerve (vagus being Latin for wandering) that we covered in chapter 5 starts at the lower skull and travels down the torso, clustering in the chest and then the gut region. This is the vagus we're getting to here.

Because the vagus has such a presence in the torso, moving your torso can have a real impact on this nerve. Simple, easy movements that stretch, lengthen, and gently twist your torso can help to apply the vagal brake. As you might remember from our previous discussion on your vagal break, it can significantly decrease your fight/flight reactivity, and significantly increase your tend/befriend and rest/digest responses. With even just a few moments of neck stretches or spinal twists, your body can become more able to call off the armed guards—and maybe even to roll out the welcome mat for the experience at hand.

It really can be only a few movements and off you go to the next thing. I have often felt like Super(wo)man ducking into a phone booth for a quick presto change-o. Superman put on his flying suit and cape, but I've been known to duck into a quiet room or corner to move my vagus: changing out of my fear reactivity, red-alert ensemble, and into a calm-alert getup that helps me feel and see more clearly. Luckily the movements I propose here aren't limited to superheroes; they can do the trick for us too. And they're not limited to phone booths. We can enjoy them from the comfort of our living rooms, our offices, even the bathroom of a stressful event. Wherever you happen to be, your vagus is there too. And for long-term investment in these personal transformation powers, these vagal-toning movements can also be a great comfort when practiced at your leisure, and at some length.

Dacher Keltner of UC Berkeley's Greater Good Science Center writes about and researches the vagus extensively. I think it is safe to say he is a big fan of the nerve. His research shows that vagal tone promotes emotion regulation and calmness and relates to prosocial behavior, which he defines as trustworthiness, empathy, and general kindness toward others *and self* (Keltner et al. 2014). Did you catch that? A nerve that helps us be less self-critical and more self-kind; what's not to like? Something as simple as moving your neck and torso can awaken what might be like a sleeping giant for you—a giant of calmness, trustworthiness, and caring.

Importantly, Keltner and his colleagues found that more and more vagal input did *not* lead to more and more stress relief. In their studies, there was a sweet spot where the gains were highest, and beyond that point, the effects lessened. They even backfired, as shown in excessive vagal braking. So too much of this good thing does *not* promote more goodness. It might even cause a braking that leaves you *under*whelmed, *un*trusting, or *dis*connected. This is further support for the "less is more and more is too much" school of thought I'm advocating in this book. Easy does it. Feel your way in. Your sensations of ease are your best guide.

Try This: Gentle Neck Stretches for Vagal Tone

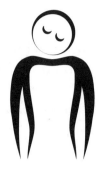 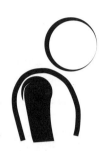

1. Sitting or standing comfortably, take a relaxing breath, then invite the muscles of your neck, shoulders, and torso to soften a bit.

2. Gently tip your head to one side, allowing your ear to ease toward your shoulder, then allow your shoulder to relax down, away from your ear. No strain at all; just let gravity assist you. Breathe into this stretch.

3. Bring your head back up to center. Take a nice slow and low breath in and out.

4. Gently tip your head over to the other side. Now allow this ear to ease toward your shoulder, and your shoulder to then soften down away from your ear on this second side. Relax your neck, creating space for your muscles to stretch.

5. Bring your head back up to center, and again take a nice slow and low breath.

6. Now tip your head gently forward toward your chest. No goal, just letting your head fall easily forward, chin softly lowering toward your chest. Easy does it. Enjoy a few long breaths in this stretch.

7. Bring your head back up to center and take a few breaths.

8. Take a look around, notice anything around you that pleases you: a view, quality of the light, an object around you.

9. Last, notice how your body feels now.

Good for you.

Movements to Soothe your System

So what movements awaken these positive powers? They're as accessible as tipping your head from side to side (a) and lowering your chin toward your chest (b), which you just did in the guided exercise. You can also add lengthening your spine to twist gently through your torso to each side (c) (see the illustrations). This is the most portable of the abracadabra vagal movements. But it's also easy to add in a full-bodied stretch up (d) and then to each side (e) if you've got a little more room. (See the Gentle Standing Stretches guide on page 151 for more guidance.) And if you have a clean floor available, and a few more minutes, your options open up considerably. You can start on your hands and knees for a little arching and curving (f), then lie on your back to pull your knees to your chest for a gentle squeeze (g), and spend a little time in a lying down twist, relaxing, breathing, or shooting the breeze (h). You can then rest for a moment on your back with your knees bent, soles of your feet on the floor (i), and finally you may want to take a few moments curled into a ball, breathing easily and enjoying a moment of turning inward (j). (See the Gentle Floor Stretches guide on page 152 for more guidance.)

The illustrations provide a visual guide to all of these movements. If you are already familiar with these movements, have at it; enjoy playing with them in a way that feels good to you. If you'd like more instruction, continue to use the neck stretches, floor stretches, and standing stretches guides in this chapter.

You can also add some long "ahhhhs" or "oohhhhhhs" to the mix; those can always enhance the benefits of your vagal efforts, because the wandering nerve is connected to your vocal cords. And if you're taking time for a longer trip to your vagus, your ears can help you out too. Music you enjoy, a podcast that relaxes you, or other sounds you like will also positively engage your vagus.

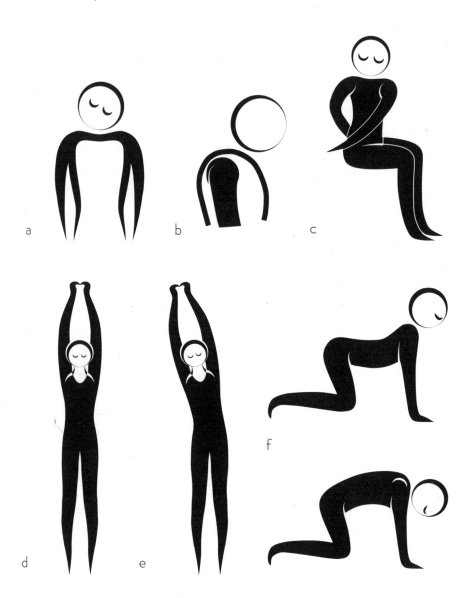

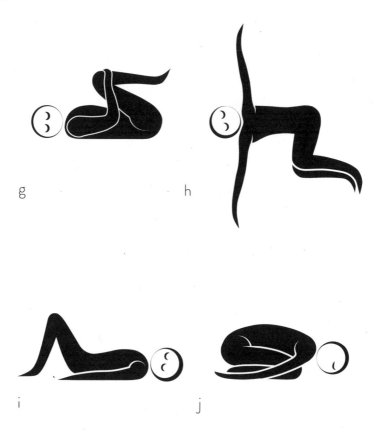

g

h

i

j

Getting to your vagus in 1, 2, 3:

1. Stretch your neck side to side or your torso in a gentle twist.

2. Add long exhales with the sound "ahhhhhhh" or "ooohhhhh."

3. Listen to soothing sounds: nature, music, a relaxing audiobook.

Vagal Science

In a study comparing yogic postures, walking in a park, and a control group doing no movement, significant *and immediate* increases in vagal tone were associated with yoga movement but *not* with walking or no movement (Khattab et al. 2007). However, the researchers found that while yoga was the only practice that immediately changed vagal tone, *both* yogic postures and walking had positive impacts on vagal tone over the course of twenty-four hours. Confirming that yoga stretches—a.k.a. postures and/or movements that target your head, chest, and pelvis—are best for immediate vagal impact, yet more general body movements like walking also have a positive *time-release* effect on our well-being nerve, the vagus, too.

General Movement Guide

The stretches shown in the figures are certainly not an exhaustive collection, but they are simple and doable for most bodies. Of course, do not do any stretches that do not feel safe for you. Also, you may know other similar movements that you want to add to this mix. Or you might use these stretches as a launching pad to discover new and different ways you like to move for the purpose of ease. If it feels relieving and soothing, you've probably involved your vagus. Get creative. Feel into it. Trust your body.

Try This: Gentle Standing Stretches for Vagal Tone

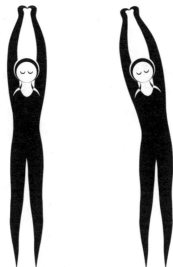

1. Standing comfortably with your feet close together, reach your arms up overhead and interlace your fingers.

2. Keeping your fingers interlaced, turn the palms of your hands up toward the ceiling and stretch up long and tall. Breathe there for a moment.

3. Next, reach your still interlaced hands, palms upward, over to the right. Lengthen up and then tip your torso over so that your left side gets very long and open.

4. Reach back up to the center, and again lengthen up, then tip over to the left. This time, lengthen your right side body, allowing your right side to lengthen and stretch.

5. Return back to the center. Release your arms to rest alongside your body and relax. Stand and breathe there for a moment.

6. Notice if there is anywhere in your body that feels some ease, relief, or even subtle okayness. Take in those sensations for a moment. Easy does it; no big deal.

Good for you!

Try This: Gentle Floor Stretches for Vagal Tone

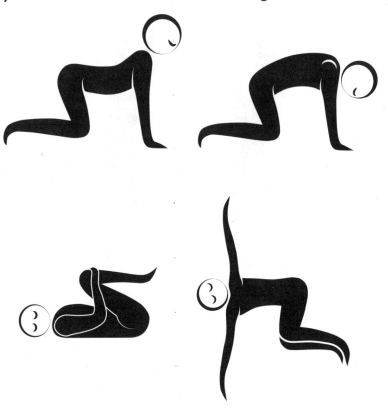

1. Start on your hands and knees, with hands vertically in line with shoulders and knees in line with hips.

2. Begin to gently arch your back so the top of your head and your tailbone are pointing up toward the ceiling while your belly curves downward.

3. Then reverse this into an opposite curve, so the top of your head and your tailbone are pointing toward the floor, while your middle back is curved up toward the ceiling.

4. Repeat a few times with long smooth breaths.

5. Now lie down on your back and gently bring your knees in toward your chest. Hug them in if it's comfortable. Take a few long breaths.

6. Bring your knees gently over to the right side of your body to rest them on the floor, and turn your head to the left. Stretch your arms out to each side like a wise letter "T." Breathe slow and low.

7. Bring your knees, one at a time, back up to your chest and then roll, shifting both knees over to the floor on your left, turning your head to the right. Arms stretched out to each side, nice and wide. Breathe slow and low.

8. Bring your knees back up to the center, one at a time. Then place the soles of your feet on the floor, a little wider apart than your hips. Let your knees fall together and rest against each other. Relax there for a moment and breathe.

9. Notice how you feel now compared to before you took this stretch break. Sense any areas of relief or ease.

Good for you!

MOVING TO THAW YOUR FREEZE

Now we come to the third option for movement to promote self-regulation: moving to thaw your freeze. The freeze state dates circa…prehistory; the ice of your freeze response just might come from the ice age. Without pinpointing exactly when this survival strategy became mainstream for our ancient ancestors, suffice it to say: evolution certainly has a hand in this mode of your reactivity. Professor, researcher, and developer of Poly Vagal Theory, Stephen Porges describes the freeze reaction as being orchestrated from within the oldest and most primitive branch of our vagus—which, yes, we have in common with the most ancient of reptiles.

The Ice Comes from Our Evolution

When our stresses overwhelm us, but taking actions to protect ourselves—flight/fight—is not an option, our evolutionary disposition slams on the brakes and moves us into a freeze. Freeze is marked by an enormous spike in sympathetic activation (the gas pedal), while at the same time adding overpowering parasympathetic activity (the brake). Press as hard as you can on the gas and brake simultaneously, and you get freeze. Think of a deer in the headlights. The deer recognizes that the car behind those oncoming headlights is much more powerful, fast, and generally intimidating than the deer herself is. The deer knows she doesn't really stand a chance in a face-off with the car. So she buries the flood of reactivity deep within her and freezes.

If you've encountered a deer in your headlights, you've probably seen there is much more going on behind those eyes than a placid stillness. Don't let that immobility masquerade as tranquility. Under that statue-like exterior is a massive surge of adrenaline and tension trapped within her muscles that will eventually need a way out of her body. In evolution's design, and in most cases activating the deer, she will have the chance to dart off the road and release all that buried reactivity to her heart's content, and to her nervous system's delight. Movement to thaw *your* freeze can be an opportunity for you to do the same as that intelligent deer after you encounter your own internal ice.

The Melt Is Mandated

Porges (1996) observes that when stress impacts your body, your vagus communicates with your primitive brain centers, directing you to either *act on* your mobilized energy or successfully *calm it*. Your vagus— the master nerve of your brainstem, heart, and gut, the longest cranial nerve in your body—wants resolution. It does not want to be caught in limbo with all that survival energy coursing through your body *without* a course of action. Nor does it want to be stuck in agitation without an eventual calming that lets the energy be put to a satisfying rest. Limbo land is terrible for your functioning. When you have a survival movement frozen within you, your whole body-mind system operates suboptimally.

Repeatedly *not* acting on your movement impulses can have serious consequences. An ongoing freeze in your vagus has been hypothesized to be a factor in diseases like chronic fatigue, irritable bowel syndrome, and obsessive-compulsive disorder. Instead of staying frozen, we can melt the internal ice by finding time, even months or years after the initial freeze occurred, to allow our physical instincts to generate physical activity, yielding to our intuitive movements. These movements are the long-awaited response that the primitive brain and the vagus had been calling for when instructing you to either truly soothe your reactivity or act on it—a.k.a. get moving!

In the preceding sections, we've discussed ways of soothing the vagus by calming your activation. Now we will take a note from that deer in the headlights who then bounds off to safety. You'll now learn ways of acting on your impulses to move after a freeze occurs. Following your instinct to move can provide deep relief within your primitive brain, vagus, and, indeed, your entire body-mind system. To explain how movement helps to melt the ice of freeze, I often share a story about my dog, Atlas. The kids I've worked with especially like it, but usually the kid in everyone can appreciate its simple modeling.

My dog Atlas is fairly little; not teacup size, but a large shoebox is pretty close; think of a snow boots size box. So when a big dog from the neighborhood passed us one day as we were setting out for a walk, Atlas froze as the large dog approached. The much bigger dog gave little Atlas a thorough sniff-down and a menacing growl or two. Not a hair on Atlas's head moved while the much bigger dog was bearing down on him. Atlas was like a statue. I know I've been there myself; probably you have, too. When fight or flight is clearly not an option because the stressor we face is overpowering, or feels overpowering, our body involuntarily goes into a freeze or shutdown.

My dog stood stock-still and looked like he was barely breathing, poor guy. This intimidation needed to come to a close quickly. The neighbor and I didn't chat, so to Atlas's relief, and mine, it was only a moment before the big dog passed. Once little Atlas could tell that the coast was clear, he set off. Running up and down the path, barking and jumping and shaking vigorously. It was, in truth, a comical sight. But also, deep evolutionary intelligence was at play right before my eyes, and I loved it. After Atlas had sufficiently released all the fear and tension he had been holding in during the inquisition, he ran right up to me and began to lick my ankles. He was back to his jovial and social self. No residue of freeze or fear remained in him because he had followed his instinctual movement cycle to its completion. His instincts had led him to freeze, wait for the threat to pass, and then let loose, doing his funky run, shake, and bark number so as to melt all that demoralizing bullying away, lest it become lodged in his being long term.

We need to take a page from the dog's (or other animal's) playbook. We need to listen to our instinctual drives and give ourselves opportunities to discharge the electrical surges that pulse through us once our survival system has been awakened. This might mean allowing your fist to freely pound on the steering wheel after another car hazardously cuts you off. It may take the form of stepping into a separate room from your partner after a shouting match and allowing your whole body to shake it all off, or maybe a kick or two to the couch (but no broken toes, please). It can also take the shape of pounding out some frustrations on a hiking trail or neighborhood jog. Stanford professor Sapolsky recommends physical activity as an active way of coping with stress and an effective way to alter our stress responses.

For one client, letting the anger from a past situation finally have time to move through and out of her body was very relieving. Gabriella had lived through a very difficult and at times shocking period with her husband. Anger coursed through her intermittently during our sessions. She felt the tension most notably in her arms and hands, and she had an urge to punch. So punching is just what we did: sometimes to the air, sometimes with resistance from one of her hands to the other, sometimes into a cushion or pillow. The punching gave her release, soothed her body-mind system, and kept her anger from bubbling up and spilling onto innocent others.

We worked with punching for several months, and with each release she felt less anger at her husband and more able to organically feel forgiveness and compassion for him. By following these instincts within the safety of therapy, she was able to release her anger to the air, a cushion, and so on, and not at work, at home, or with strangers who happened to pass by at the wrong moment. Little by little, over time, she felt the release of the anger, the return of her hard-won well-being, and a true recovery from what had seemed like an insurmountable chasm in her marriage.

Big and Small Movements Can Have a Big Impact

In addition to big movements to assist our own stress recovery, we can also benefit enormously from physicality that is much subtler. It can be as unassuming as giving your body time and space for hardly perceivable trembling, which often happens when a long-held stress reaction is finally being released. Such a subtle yet deeply affecting bodily release occurred during a conversation I had with a young woman as she was getting a long-held burden off her chest.

Charlotte and I hadn't seen each other in years; in fact, not since her young teen years when she had been a regular in some of my classes. She reached out one day to reconnect, and we were able to spend a lovely few hours together catching up. Near the end of our time together, our conversation came around to a serious incident she had confided in me about when she was a young girl. I was careful to gently inquire about it so as not to alarm or upset her. Charlotte did recall confiding in me so many years ago, but she'd forgotten all about it until we met again that afternoon.

It turned out she had greatly embellished the scenario she'd shared with me some eight years prior. I wasn't put off by this at all. I know young minds are given to being emphatic. I was actually relieved that her original story was not entirely true. I told her so. She revealed some of the shame and guilt she'd felt about having told that tale to me all those years ago. With my empathy and support for Charlotte and my understanding of her embellishment, she began to tremble and described to me what she was noticing in her body. I explained that her trembling could be a sign of healthy release, her body seizing this opportunity to melt the freeze state that accompanied the original tall tale telling so many years ago.

This seemed likely to her, and she allowed this gentle trembling to run its course, giving her body time and space to unwind. She felt some of the knots of guilt and shame she'd been holding about her youthful deception slowly releasing. She continued to allow her sensations and to comment intermittently on what she was noticing. After a few minutes, Charlotte said she was feeling better, more present and comfortable in our conversation once again. It seemed to both of us, but most importantly to her, that the past was the past, and that her schoolgirl exaggeration was understandable and completely forgivable. Her body released the freeze, and then her mind followed with new perspectives. Self-judgment was giving way to self-understanding via a gentle wave of muscle contractions and releases, culminating in ease.

Try This

Letting Your Body Thaw from Freeze

We cannot schedule time for melting our stored reactivity. Unfortunately, we can't direct our muscles to tremble away our historical stresses on cue. However, we *can* be like Atlas and seize opportunities to shake it off when they present themselves. Or be like Charlotte and allow subtle trembling to run its course once it arises naturally on its own. And be like Gabriella and allow ourselves time and a safe place to punch (or stomp, or kick) when such an urge arises.

With what you now know about thawing your freeze, be on the lookout for moments in which your body needs a little support to complete an instinct. Recognize moments that are twitchy, trembly, or fidgety. See what happens if you bring kind awareness to these sensations. Witness what transpires next if you allow these movements to occur; to move through you and then out of you.

Feeling the result of your movement is essential. The awareness of the release, or shift, or completion (even partial completion) is what aids your thaw.

Remember, easy does it. Less is more. Good for you!

Shame Is Often as Cold as Ice

When shame lays itself over your stress events like a blanket, freeze can all too easily overtake your system. When your thoughts, feelings, or actions are deemed unacceptable or impermissible, they can become held captive within you. Both Gabriella and Charlotte were struggling under the weight of shame. Coming out from under it was part of what allowed their physical discharge to occur. If shame is infesting your own stress memories, it can be helpful to acknowledge the evolutionary role it played for our ancestors and the importance of thawing. Shame can creep into many circumstances. It is wise to keep an eye out for it.

Shame found its way into Charlotte when she judged her teenage embellishments as unacceptable. It found its way into Gabriella through the societal "shoulds" of marriage, and the widespread falsehood that everything is going well at the Johnsons' house, so why is my household struggling? Another example of shame interrupting recovery processes comes from a great tragedy and increasing reality that touched the life of my client Shauna: school gun violence. In this case, the shame surrounding the reactivity was frozen as solidly as the reactivity itself.

A staff member at a college that had suffered a campus shooting confided in Shauna, explaining that one of the most difficult parts of the recovery process for the students at her college was the way students were rushed into praying for the shooter, finding compassion and forgiveness for him, and not really receiving any support for feeling scared or angry. Being encouraged to deny their anger and replace it with immediate compassion left many feeling ashamed for what is a natural response to senseless violence: outrage. Unfortunately, sidestepping fear and anger neither erases it nor soothes it. On the contrary, it may well lodge it more deeply into a person's system without a healthy means of exit, while leaving shame in the role of holding in feelings that needn't be impermissible in the first place.

Circumstances like these are prime opportunities for allowing movement, subtle or overt, to cycle through you and out of you. This is entirely different from *acting* on our impulses. Movement for stress resilience does *not* involve engaging in acts of violence. Movement for stress resilience is allowing your body to *feel* the fear or anger or grief that is right there beneath the surface and give it a moment to move through you and *out of you*, little by little. For example, the fear might crave putting your hand up to block your face. The anger might want to push or kick. The grief may need to be softly held or wrapped in a cozy sweater. These are all sensations that can be safely allowed, *without* hurting anyone. When these impulses are allowed in appropriate situations, like in the quiet of your home, or the support of a somatic therapist's office, or the safety of a hike in nature, they can come to completion and then *exit your body*.

If we shame ourselves into sidestepping or dismissing our "messy" primitive reactions, we are effectively making a nice place for them to move in and set up long-term living arrangements inside of us. By *not* allowing ourselves to express feelings like anger, fear, or grief, they become *more* prominent in our body-mind. Rushing toward forgiveness and empathy sidelines our evolutionarily based body-mind recovery. If, instead, we find healthy outlets for our primitive responses through the movement suggested in this chapter, and with imagery from chapter 6, we will very likely help the states of empathy and understanding to blossom from within us, rather than forcing ourselves to lay them on top of our pain.

Supporting Your Primitive Brain Through Fear, Anger, or Grief

Giving yourself this kind of support is a deeply personal process, one that you will need to play with as you find your way. If recurring sensations seem to nag at you, listen to them. Clues can be seen in feeling quick flashes of physical aggression, or seeming to fall inexplicably into the felt sense of grief; perhaps your body often repeats fear reactivity with intense heat, constriction, or numbness.

Experiment with allowing your instincts to guide you to react, bringing your reactions *to inanimate objects in a safe environment.*

What if you let yourself respond to the fear within the protection of your home? Or let your body stomp out some feelings on a hike in nature? Perhaps you would feel some relief to wrap yourself up in a blanket and provide some holding to the grief or sadness within.

Sometimes the movements are much more subtle and occur much more at the level of sensation than of action. Allow your tissues to guide you to micro-movements of release—cycles of tension and release; fluctuations of heat, then cold; or subtle vibrations moving through you.

Remember: easy does it, less is more. Good for you.

THE RELIEF OF MOVEMENT

Giving our bodies time and space to discharge long-held tensions can be deeply healing for all of us. If a memory is frozen in your tissues, movement can help the stress imprint melt. Whether you follow a subtle or gross muscular impulse is up to your unique needs. Releases can range from very subtle shifts in your muscles, tendons, or bones, to large expressions like squeezing, running, or punching—in safe, nonharming ways. Listen to your instincts, and if the impulse is hard to decipher, why not try both and sense which feels more relieving to you?

As your body moves out of the holding pattern it froze into during your historic stress event, new freedoms can be felt from the inside out. These freedoms are the building blocks of your resilience pathways. These pathways build the all-important body intelligence of how to get back out of your stress reactivity. Resilience of this sort may help James Joyce's Mr. Duffy to no longer live a short distance from his body, but to reinhabit himself once again. How close to your body do you live now? How close to your body would you like to live?

Learning the language of your body takes time, patience, and practice, but it can certainly be done. Listening to your subtle physical needs, your wants, and your sensitivities will serve you well on your path toward somatic regulation. Whether you're setting aside time to move for soothing, move for your vagus, or move to thaw freeze, your unique map and directions will be within you and for you. The tools in this chapter will help you find your way. And remember: follow the sensations of relief, look for the experience of feeling safe, and trust your muscles to lead the way.

CHAPTER 8

At Home in You

We arrive at the end of this book, and at the beginning of a new leg of this journey: your ongoing journey of your ongoing well-being. The task now is to gather all the pieces of this book that feel most relevant to you and to adapt them to feel custom-made *for you*. We all know the expression "toe the line." Well, when it comes to self-regulation, resilience, and embodied experiences of safety and ease, toeing lines is not what's called for. For this leg of your journey, it's all about you. These tools are for you; they have to be in service of you, tailored to you, and your skilled body-mind awareness is the best way to find just the right fit. The right fit will *feel* better; an embodied experience of well-being will begin to arise from within you. Embodied well-being and reliable self-regulation tools help you get back out from under the strain of stress. Back to safety, aliveness, and ease.

From within our own intimate understanding of our own stress and dysregulation, we can develop an equally personal knowledge of our own resilience and our returns to regulation. With this strong self-awareness—a *somatic* awareness—we each can develop the self-efficacy and agency we need to put ourselves back at the helm of our well-being. When we have custom-fitted tools at the ready, we don't have to feel stuck in activation; we know there *are* ways to get back out. As we feel our way back out of extreme stress, we begin to experience our own strength, have confidence in our skills, and feel empowered to call on our self-regulatory capacities when our nervous system calls out for help. Feeling strong and empowered helps us return to a *felt sense* of agency reclaiming an often long-lost vitality, and ultimately restoring trust in ourselves and trust in our ability to feel resilient with what life brings.

MIND AND BODY TASK

I hope this book has clearly conveyed to you that the way back out of extreme stress is a mind *and body* task. It's important to remember that our culture has long glorified the power of the mind as superior to the power of the body, *and* we have confined our smarts to our heads. The science of somatic regulation included in and beyond this book shows us it is high time we glory in the power of the body along with the mind, and expand our view of intelligence to include our highly adept gut and heart centers—as well as the cleverness found upstairs inside the skull.

> The tools in this book, and in the larger field of somatic regulation, unify your body and mind as tethered vessels in which ease, wellness, vitality, and relief can be nurtured to grow.

Building and shoring up the pathways that lead to balance and well-being requires us to learn the language of *our own* nervous system; your own system that elegantly joins your body and mind into *one whole*. Each of us is one complex, intricate, delicate, and totally interconnected body *and* mind. We are not parts; we are whole.

USE YOUR WHOLE TOOL KIT FOR YOUR WHOLE SELF

Developing personalized tools for your intricate and beautifully complex self is not a one problem, one tool situation. We each need a varied tool kit. We each benefit from a set of tools that can be used each on their own but also can and should be used in conjunction with one another. You'll find there are times when one tool or somatic skill alone does not soothe your system in the way you need; you'll need to apply two, three, or more tools one after the other, or all together, to help yourself get back out of the stress reaction that's gotten hold of you.

Have you ever needed to repair something in your home, gone to grab a tool, rummaged through your tool kit, and returned to your repair work only to find that in the end you needed a different tool? It was not until you had several tools laid out in front of you that finally you were able to settle into your task to mend or fix your broken parts. The tools in this book are much the same. It can be really helpful to metaphorically lay all your tools out in front of you when stress presents itself. Pick up one or two at a time, or one for a brief moment and then another for a while. Keep asking your *felt sense of stress* what kind of help it needs to return to a *felt sense of safety* and relief.

For example, you might feel relief if you combine a few rhythmic breaths along with some simple neck stretches. Maybe you'd follow this with a brief moment of letting your mind's eye see a reassuring image of support or protection. Perhaps on another occasion, you take a moment to see something pleasing or comforting in the environment around you, while also sensing what is okay inside you. Then further assist your regulation with a few long sighing breaths of "aaahhhs" or "ooohhhs" that vibrate all the way down to your belly. The possibilities are abundant, and there is no wrong way to combine these tools. If your body is telling you it likes that particular way you're helping yourself back out of stress, go with that. Remember, the brain isn't the only valuable decision maker here; your body has a tremendous amount of intelligence too. As was introduced in chapters 2 and 3, when it comes to extreme stress, we usually need to communicate with our primitive brain, the one that speaks in sensations, rather than the very verbal front brain. We can each use the *custom-made* combinations of self-regulation skills that bring relief to our own mind *and* body.

For those of us who find that our body-mind systems are just very good at stress, several tools administered together might be just what our resilience calls for. An example of applying several tools during a particularly challenging stress event happened quite naturally between Leah and her friend, two women both very well-versed in their own somatic-resilience tool kits.

Tears were streaming down Leah's face as she walked down the sidewalk. She was in an unfamiliar part of the city, not sure exactly where she was, and she wasn't having any luck finding the group of friends she was supposed to meet in that area. Old stress events from years past merged with the stress of that day, creating a huge storm of reactivity inside Leah's whole body-mind system. She was hot, her heart was pounding, her stomach ached, and she felt alone, scared, and overwhelmed.

After what seemed like much too long to her, but was probably just ten or so minutes, Leah was able to reach one of her friends by cell phone. Leah and her friend figured out that they were only a few blocks apart. Still Leah's overwhelm came pouring out through gasps and tears, and Leah asked her friend to meet her on the nearest street corner, where her friend could help her navigate to the restaurant. The presence of a good friend would also help Leah journey through the stress reaction that was churning through her body-mind.

With all of her tools metaphorically laid out in front of her, Leah began to select which tool to use and when. The first tool Leah picked up that day was *seeing safety*. Having skillfully practiced seeing safety so many times before, Leah knew to guide herself to watch her friend walking down the sidewalk right toward her, a very pleasing sight at that moment; she took it in and felt its impact as much as possible. This brought a little relief and lessened her feeling of aloneness and overall activation. Next, Leah intentionally *felt her body receive* the hug she and her friend shared upon meeting up and consciously let herself feel the dose of comfort their contact offered her. She noticed her heart slowing down, sensed a little ease growing in her chest, and then felt a few deeper breaths make themselves available to her.

Leah then applied her third tool; taking advantage of the fact that her ribcage was unclenching around her lungs, she guided herself to enjoy a few more *full breaths* in and out, internally tracking the soothing effects of each breath. With increased self-regulation coming online in her nervous system, her body began to discharge some of the bodily contractions that accompany panic for her (and for many of us). She *let her body shake* off some of the tension that had seized her when she was somewhat lost and unable to find her friends in a few little shudders and some subtle trembling. She felt more relief, and her sense of ease expanded. Leah could sense that the volume in her fear brain and body had been turned down significantly. With this quieting in her fear-driven body and mind, as she and her friend began to walk to the restaurant together, she brought her attention outside of herself and began to *take notice* of the early spring flowers in some of the shop window boxes. Leah noticed how much better she now felt. The storm had passed, and she felt her resilience; most importantly, she now knew she was okay.

Leah's recovery was a steady stream of attending to her self-regulation and using stress-resilience tools in tandem. First, she used seeing: taking in the image of her friend walking toward her. Second, she used sensing: feeling the support of a hug and the subsequent relief in her body. Third, she used breathing: following her own spontaneous deeper breaths, and then inviting a few more in and out. Fourth, she used movement: shaking off some of the tension that had clutched at her arms, legs, shoulders, and back. Fifth and last, she returned to seeing: taking in some of the beauty in her immediate environment by noticing a few blossoms nearby.

Maybe this sounds like a lot of steps, but the body learns them quite naturally. Our body wants access to its own ease and well-being. The access to a recovery like Leah had comes from imprinting the process of self-regulation. Embodying your small and large successes with resilience and stress recovery *is* your imprinting. The practice of using your tools is the process of embodying your resilience and stress recovery.

> *Embodying* your return to well-being creates an imprint of self-regulation.
>
> *Imprints* become a map for your body-mind to follow when you need to get back out of stress.

At first we will need to think our way through the application of each skill. There is a phase of deciding mentally which tool to try and cognitively navigating how to use it. However, with practice, these can and do become natural and reflexive responses to stress. Over time, they can become the body's own next step after stress, a *learned* response to the *automatic* reactions that stress brings. In acquiring these skills, we are *voluntarily* imprinting regulating habits to counteract the *involuntarily* imprinted dysregulating habits our survival system has developed (whether we wanted them or not).

PRACTICE BECOMES HABIT

When working with groups, I often say that embodying regulating habits is like embodying the skills of riding a bike. At first it is a somewhat clunky and often very mentally led process. But over time, it can become quite graceful, and eventually it happens without much mental effort at all. This process played out in front of me when I helped my daughter transition from pedal brakes to hand brakes on her assent along the hierarchy of two wheeled adventure conveyance.

My daughter had become quite a proficient rider with her pedal brakes bike. You know the ones—you push backward on your pedals to stop and push forward on the pedals to go. Most of us started out on this style of bike and at some point transitioned to a bike with hand brakes. On a hand brake bike, when you pedal backward, your feet just spin in a circle while your bike continues to cruise along without any significant slowing taking place.

This feeling of spinning her feet backward, circling around and around, was alarming for my little one, especially because what she was trying to do was slow down and then stop, and spinning pedals while maintaining full cruising speed was anything but her desired outcome. But pushing her feet backward to stop had become a deeply ingrained habit—a somatic imprint of sorts. So in her first days of transitioning to her new wheels I ran alongside her bike, coaching her into a new bodily reaction—developing a new imprint. Her old impulse was a desire to stop, then push her *feet* backward. Her new reaction needed to be a desire to stop, then squeeze the hand brake levers *with her hands*. Replace feet with hands. Seems easy enough.

So along a flat stretch we would go, her pedaling, me jogging alongside. And when I saw her feet spinning in a backward circle—and a little alarm in her eyes—I would call out, "Squeeze with your hands, squeeze with your hands." She would, thus slowing down and replacing alarm with pleasure. It was a somewhat clunky process, but the new skills were being acquired. In time, my verbal cues were abbreviated to "Squeeze hands" and finally just "hands." And little by little she transitioned, as all bike riders do, from being instructed *from the outside* to use her hand brakes, to instructing herself *from the inside* to use her hand brakes. First instructions in this case, the external ones, came from yours truly, then internal instructions from herself, and eventually she just *automatically* used her hand brakes whenever she wanted to slow or stop.

Can you imagine a world where we all needed ongoing outside coaching every time we wanted to come to a complete and full stop?! Thankfully, that is *not* necessary. This process of internalizing and automatizing our responses is something we can each do with not just our bikes, but also our stress resilience and reset skills. First, we'll follow *instructions from the outside,* then we'll follow *instructions from inside,* and over time these resilience pathways will become our individual and uniquely tailored *automatic response* to stress. This newly imprinted action becomes an entirely new stress response, a *positive feedback loop.* A loop that often starts out a little bumpy, as in Leah's case, but can then be soothed and relieved with some attention and care. This kind of loop goes something like the figure here.

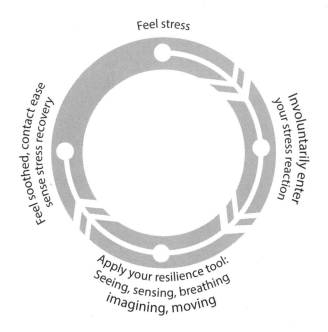

Feel stress

Involuntarily enter your stress reaction

Apply your resilience tool: Seeing, sensing, breathing, imagining, moving

Feel soothed, contact ease sense stress recovery

Periods of extreme stress can leave your system very good at stress reactivity and her sister, dysregulation. In times like these, you may have a lot of negative feedback, or unwanted reactivity, looping inside you. But you *can* reassign those feedback loops to become good at stress resilience and *returning to regulation.* This will develop positive feedback and desired reactivity and responsiveness looping inside you. You can do this. It really does work.

Coaching Yourself

To create these positive loops, first you metaphorically run alongside yourself and give *external cues.* Maybe you set smartphone reminders to practice these skills, or you set aside some time in your day's agenda to practice your tools, or you find a certain place where you curl up with this book and go through the exercises. You can also develop places for mini practice sessions, such as a free moment at a stop light, a few minutes of a hike you're on, or that quiet time before you fall asleep at night.

Next, your positive loops begin to occur with more subtle *internal cues:* you mentally remind yourself to practice some seeing and sensing after you are startled by running into a foe at the local coffee shop. You guide yourself through some rhythmic breathing after you find yourself awake and worrying in the middle of the night. You might spend time with some regulating imagery after an upsetting event keeps replaying in your mind. Maybe after a stressful phone call, you take time for a few easy stretches that soothe your system.

Finally, these positive loops become *automatic responses.* Your breathing automatically deepens after the trigger has passed. Your eyes seek out pleasing or even just neutral views after you-know-who leaves your office. Your neck draws itself into a simple side-to-side stretch with a few "ahhhhs" or "ooooohhhs" after you've sent a difficult email. You find yourself developing a soothing version of the internal movie that has been playing in your mind and creating agitation.

Developing New Imprints

- Externally cued responses

- Internally cued responses

- Automatically cued responses

Coaching Comes from Within

Once these regulating imprints become strong, you can sometimes find yourself simply allowing your tools to do their thing in your body-mind after a stress event takes place. I was amazed to see my tools take care of my return to regulation after a very close call on a snow-covered highway.

We were on a family trip, two parents in front, two kids in back, slowly motoring up a two-lane mountain highway, traveling east toward the mountains at an elevation of 6,000 feet above sea level. The roads were blanketed in several inches of snow. Our snow tires and four-wheel drive were holding out pretty well thus far. Then all of a sudden our car began to spin out of control. In a span of 30 to 45 seconds, our truck 180-ed itself, leaving us facing west and on the opposite side of our two-lane road. At least we were pointing to right direction for the flow of traffic! As we spun, I watched my body react first with flight instincts. I had a split-second impulse to jump out of the car. Luckily that was completely halted by my logical brain recognizing that the car was careening in such a way that any attempt to flee would result in my being run over by our vehicle.

Then came the fight response, and I had a momentary impulse to yell out some kind of command—to someone, anyone—but I don't know anything about driving in the snow, which was why I wasn't driving, so calling out seemed unwise. Next, my arms threw themselves up in the air and froze still in a strange position like they were goalposts for a football game, my fingertips grazing the interior roof of our car. My eyes felt stuck wide open, staring at the twelve-foot-tall snow bank we were headed toward. Once the car was still, our skid complete and with no collision having occurred, our skillful driver—my husband—drove us slowly and safely to where we could get turned around to once again face east toward our original destination and on the proper side of the road. We parked safely on the shoulder. In that moment, I loved that shoulder like I never had loved another.

I momentarily felt a rush of nausea, and for a split second thought I might throw up, the intelligent gut vagus talking to me ("Clear the decks and toss any excess baggage overboard!"). I recognized just how much fear was coursing through my body. We all started talking at once, simultaneously declaring our utter gladness to be safe and snapshots of what we each had going on inside of us as we were skidding just moments before. This kind of social engagement is the first adaptive move of the smart vagus nerve, soothing our nervous systems with the vibrations of our voices, experiencing the relief produced by our smile muscles, and our ears taking in the joy and safe connections with others who are near and dear, all of which contribute to powerful vagal braking. None of us internally asked ourselves to do this; we just did it, thanks to well-imprinted resilience pathways.

I then began to instinctively breathe rhythmically, elongating my exhales. Again, this was not a conscious decision; my lungs just started to do this for me. Thank you, lungs, for these rhythmic breaths! Next, I watched myself scan the snow-covered environment, taking notice of how lucky we had been that during our entire 360 (half of it skid-powered, half of it motor-powered) we had been the only car on the road for that entire span of time and the two minutes or so following. Thank you, eyes, for recognizing safety. Then I noticed my legs were trembling, and I said out loud, "I'm shaking," to no one in particular, just an instinct to give this important event time and space. I internally congratulated my legs and let them subtly tremble; meanwhile, my arms were finally relaxing from their goal-post position. Thank you, legs and arms, for discharging all that fear and freeze reactivity. Then my mind began playing the clip of our skid toward the snow bank and seemed to zoom in on the *not* hitting the bank part—rewinding and replaying it a few more times. And my internal moviemaker enjoyed drawing out the safe return to the east-facing side of the road and that glorious quiet and still shoulder of the road we were parked on. Thank you, mental film crew: that movie was Oscar-worthy for me. I wasn't so much asking my body or mind to do these things as I was giving my body and mind time and space to do these things for itself. That's the pathways making use of their own skills: resilience, resilience, resilience. Thank you, resilience pathways: job well done.

This was truly a great relief on so many levels. Not only were we safe, but I felt really powerful and really proud of my body-mind system. You can do this too. Really, you can.

And, it's really important to acknowledge that it's not always as simple as steps one, two, and three. Sometimes we find ourselves in a tangled web of stress reaction on top of stress reaction, on top of trauma, on top of more traumas, and while this tool kit is potent, it will not be enough for every situation. There are definitely situations for which you'll need more tools, more help, and more guidance than this book can provide.

WHEN TO CALL FOR ADDITIONAL SUPPORT

Returning to regulation is not always a solo journey. In fact, often we need trusted companions along for some of the ride. While we really can facilitate true relief and resilience for ourselves, there are also times when we need the guidance of a skilled advisor. When those times come, a skilled somatic practitioner will counsel you in the use of these and additional tools that will effectively address the causes and symptoms of your unique dysregulation.

But how to know when to go it alone and when to call for aid? I recommend returning to the 1 to 10 scale from chapter 2, where 1 = mild stress, 5 = moderate stress, and 10 = extreme stress. With a stress level that hovers between 1 and 5 on this scale, you are very likely to feel effective in mitigating your reactivity on your own. In these cases, crack open this book, refresh your memory, and remind your body about its self-regulation capacities.

When your stress hovers between 5 and 6 regularly, it's important to shore up your support system. Make sure you are connecting with trusted friends and/or family and getting support with your stress resilience in addition to working with the tools found here. Maybe you form a book group with this book, sharing tales of your resilience successes, and opening up with safe others about the real and human experiences that happen along the way. In this situation, it can also be helpful to seek support from a somatic specialist either from time to time or more regularly if possible.

If your stress level is persistently 7 to 10, do all you can to get professional support in addition to using the tools in this book. Seek out a skilled somatic therapist with whom you feel safe and understood. Work with this professional on the underlying stress imprints that are affecting you, along with developing the skills and embodying the tools in this book to support your somatic therapy. This is certainly a both/and situation, not an either/or: therapy *and* these self-regulation skills, not one or the other.

There is no need to go it alone. Our nervous systems are designed to coregulate—regulate with each other. We have evolved as beings that need to receive and give regulation support to one another regularly, consistently, and dependably. As the old Barbra Streisand song goes, "People who need people are the luckiest people in the world." If you know you would benefit from more support, seek it out, prioritize it, and get your nervous system the help it needs—the help you need, the support you deserve.

OPTIMAL ACTIVATION

With a nurtured and strengthened body-mind stress release system, and confidence in your abilities to self-regulate, you get a huge prize: to be here, engaged in your life, feeling connected and safe. For all of us, engagement, connection, and safety is a continuum. We move around on it and feel sometimes more, sometimes less engaged or safe or connected. This is natural; this happens to all of us.

We can picture the range of engagement, connection, safety, and overall regulation in three zones: middle zone, high zone, and low zone. In the center of our middle zone we have optimal activation, in which we are calm, alert, engaged, and optimally regulated. We can also tolerably dip or rise into engagement that is somewhat outside of optimal but where we are still highly functional and mostly regulated: our functional-activation zones. When our reactivity is far outside of this middle zone, we can rise too high and become hyperactivated, or the inverse, when we can dip too low below our functional range and we become hypoactivated. Chapters 1 and 2 discuss hyper- and hypoactivation further, if you'd like to refresh your memory.

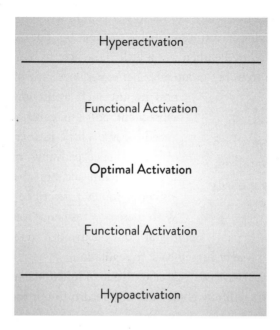

LEAVING OPTIMAL

We are all going to leave the optimal range, not just occasionally, but regularly. Moving out of our peak range is a normal and ongoing part of being human. In addition, we will also leave our functional-activation range when stresses are too high or too frequent. Yet there is good news: *we can get back.* In fact, every return is an important victory for your nervous system. Having skills and knowledge to guide yourself back to functionality and into your own optimal zone again *is* the process of resilience. Also, returning from hyper- and hypoactivation skillfully can expand your functional zone, making it more possible for you to work through stresses that previously would have overwhelmed you—that would have taken you way out of your range and kept you there. But with practice, you'll be able to get back.

Increasing one's range can mean you gain function in areas of your life where previously you were unable to function. For example, Leah, whose story I relayed earlier, was a little more able to handle being lost and separated from her group after her experience returning to regulation in just such a circumstance. Every subsequent return to regulation she experienced became a little further development of her resilience pathways, away from her stress autobahn and onto her newly built resilience routes I described in chapter 1. With these new resilience routes, her functional zones expanded more and more each time she brought herself back to regulation.

> We're not trying to keep ourselves from moving into states of activation; rather, we are increasing our ability to come back from them.

If we find ourselves outside of our zone of functional activation and use our tools to skillfully come back and return to our functional zone once again, our nervous system gains confidence in its ability to deal with similar kinds of activation the next time. Over time, your system will incorporate these experiences of activation into its functional capacity. Bit by bit, your functional range continues to grow as your ability to *come back from activation* increases. Embodied stress resilience becomes the norm, not the exception, and you find yourself able to truly thrive in more and more aspects of your life. Engaged. Connected. Safe.

A FULL LIFE

Activation is part of a full life, but it does not have to overshadow all the other parts of your life. For people who have lived with extreme stress, the feeling that stress reactivity is ruling their life is common. The power to recognize and to help soothe our own states of activation can be truly transformative, tremendously empowering, and deeply relieving. Agency and feelings of self-efficacy with stress resilience have a tremendous positive impact on our experiences of ourselves and of the world around us; the world within and the world around become much more welcoming places to be.

Newfound resilience pathways not only return you to healthy states of regulation but also help you to be able to *do* what you didn't before, to *say* what you couldn't before, and to *be* where you weren't before. Access to stress resilience makes the world a much more vivid and inviting place to live. To be able to *be*, to *say*, and to *do* these newly appealing things while simultaneously feeling your own experience of regulation, wellness, and ease is to live in this vivid world right from *within your body*—not the short distance that James Joyce's Mr. Duffy was stuck with. Instead of distance, we find ourselves happily close to the aliveness, tenderness, connection, and surprises life brings.

Being able to apply tools that help you bring yourself back from stress triggers places you in the safety of your own skilled care. Your whole body-mind system comes to know its capacities to recover from stress and its own pathways of resilience. Our beautiful and complex nervous systems need not run us headlong into ongoing stress reactivity nor let evolution convince us that danger lurks close by. We do have the ability to reassure our survival brain. We are capable of relieving our vigilant body. We can learn how to recognize and internalize the care, protection, and basic safety that we need, that every body-mind needs—and that every body-mind deserves. We can connect with the world within us and around us, feeling at home in ourselves and at home with each other. And to paraphrase a poetic passage that has whispered itself to me over so many years, we can sit down in the warm lap of our own skin and know that we are okay.

> When you can apply tools that help you bring yourself back from the pain and stress of anxiety and overwhelm, you are in the safety of your own skilled care.

Acknowledgments

There are so many people to thank. Although this book has one author, there are dozens of people standing beside me who have each helped to give rise to this work. I am so grateful to my teachers, mentors, and colleagues who have explored, explained, and experienced this important work alongside me. I am so indebted to great thinkers like Levine, van der Kolk, and Porges, without whom I would not have even known I could investigate and research; and, of course, to the Somatic Experiencing Training Institute which provides such excellent therapeutic training and wisdom. To each person I have had the privilege to support and to learn from, and who have helped to deepen this research, thank you. I cannot even name all the many colleagues and friends who read these chapters, offering ideas, insights, and all-important interest in these pages, especially everyone at New Harbinger. Special thanks to Mel and Manu, my fellow travelers on this journey; your support was essential. To my husband for encouraging me, and of course to my two daughters, who inspire me every day to keep going, learn more, and contribute.

References

Beard, C., and N. Amir, 2010. "Negative Interpretation Bias Mediates the Effect of Social Anxiety on State Anxiety." *Cognitive Therapy and Research* 34(3): 292–296.

Björkstrand, J., T. Agren, A. Frick, J. Engman, E. M. Larsson, T. Furmark, and M. Fredrikson. 2015. "Disruption of Memory Reconsolidation Erases a Fear Memory Trace in the Human Amygdala: An 18-Month Follow-Up." *PLOS ONE* 10(7): e0129393.

Brown, B. 2010. *The Gifts of Imperfection: Let Go of Who You Think You're Supposed to Be and Embrace Who You Are*, narrated by Lauren Fortgang. Audible Studios.

Goodwin, H., C. Eagleson, A. Mathews, J. Yiend, and C. Hirsch. 2016. "Automaticity of Attentional Bias to Threat in High and Low Worriers." *Cognitive Therapy and Research* 41(3): 479–488. doi:10.1007/s10608-016-9818-5

Grossi, D., M. Longarzo, M. Quarantelli, E. Salvatore, C. Cavaliere, P. De Luca, L. Trojano, and M. Aiello. 2017. "Altered Functional Connectivity of Interoception in Illness Anxiety Disorder." *Cortex* 86. 10.1016/j.cortex.2016.10.018.

Gusnard, D. A., E. Akbudak, G. L. Shulman, and M. E. Raichle. 2001. "Medial Prefrontal Cortex and Self-Referential Mental Activity: Relation to a Default Mode of Brain Function." *Proceedings of the National Academy of Sciences* 98(7): 4259–4264; doi:10.1073/pnas.071043098

Heuman, L. 2014. "Don't Believe the Hype." *Tricycle, The Buddhist Review* (October 1), https://tricycle.org/trikedaily/dont-believe-hype/.

Hirsch, C. R., and A. Mathews. 2012. "A Cognitive Model of Pathological Worry." *Behaviour Research and Therapy* 50(10): 636–646. doi:10.1016/j.brat.2012.06.007

Karavidas, M. K., P. M. Lehrer, E. Vaschillo, B. Vaschillo, H. Marin, S. Buyske,... A. Hassett. 2007. "Preliminary Results of an Open Label Study of Heart Rate Variability Biofeedback for the Treatment of Major Depression." *Applied Psychophysiology and Biofeedback* 32(1): 19–30.

Keltner, D., A. Kogan, C. Oveis, E. W. Carr, J. Gruber, I. B. Mauss, and A. Shallcross. 2014. "Vagal Activity Is Quadratically Related to Prosocial Traits, Prosocial Emotions, and Observer Perceptions of Prosociality." *Journal of Personality and Social Psychology* 107(6): 1051–1063.

Khattab, K., A. A. Khattab, J. Ortak, G. Richardt, and H. Bonnemeier. 2007. "Iyengar Yoga Increases Cardiac Parasympathetic Nervous Modulation Among Healthy Yoga Practitioners." *Evidence-Based Complementary and Alternative Medicine* 4(4): 511–517.

Lagos, L., E. Vaschillo, B. Vaschillo, P. Lehrer, M. Bates, and R. Pandina. 2008. "Heart Rate Variability Biofeedback as a Strategy for Dealing with Competitive Anxiety: A Case Study." *Biofeedback* 36(3): 109.

Lehrer, P. M., and R. Gevirtz (2014). "Heart Rate Variability Biofeedback: How and Why Does It Work?" *Frontiers in Psychology* 5, 756. doi:10.3389/fpsyg.2014.00756

Levine, P. A. 1997. *Waking the Tiger: Healing Trauma: The Innate Capacity to Transform Overwhelming Experiences.* Berkeley, CA: North Atlantic Books.

Levine, P. A. 2010. *In an unspoken voice: How the body releases trauma and restores goodness.* Berkeley, CA: North Atlantic Books.

Loftus, E. F., and J. E. Pickrell. 1995. "The Formation of False Memories." *Psychiatric Annals* 25(12): 720–725.

Loftus, E. F. 2005. "Planting Misinformation in the Human Mind: A 30-Year Investigation of the Malleability of Memory." *Learning & Memory* 12(4): 361–366.

Mogg, K., B. P. Bradley, R. Williams, and A. Mathews. 1993. "Subliminal Processing of Emotional Information in Anxiety and Depression." *Journal of Abnormal Psychology* 102(2): 304.

Netz, Y., and R. Lidor. 2003. "Mood Alterations in Mindful Versus Aerobic Exercise Modes." *Journal of Psychology* 137: 405–419. doi: 10.1080/00223980309600624

Porges, S. 1996. "Physiological Regulation in High-Risk Infants: A Model for Assessment and Potential Intervention." *Development and Psychopathology* 8(1): 43–58. doi:10.1017/S0954579400006969

Porges, S. [NICABM]. 2014. *Trauma 2014 Porges.* [Video File].

Prinsloo, G. E., H. L. Rauch, M. I. Lambert, F. Muench, T. D. Noakes, and W. E. Derman. 2011. "The Effect of Short Duration Heart Rate Variability (HRV) Biofeedback on Cognitive Performance During Laboratory Induced Cognitive Stress." *Applied Cognitive Psychology* 25, 792–801. doi: org/10.1002/acp.1750

Sapolsky, R. M. 2004. *Why Zebras Don't Get Ulcers.* New York: Owl Book/Henry Holt and Co.

Serpa, J. G., S. Taylor, and K. Tillisch. 2014. "Mindfulness-based Stress Reduction (MBSR) Reduces Anxiety, Depression, and Suicidal Ideation in Veterans." *Medical Care* 52 Suppl 5. doi:10.1097/MLR.0000000000000202

Schwerdtfeger, A. R., and A.K.S. Gerteis. 2014. "The Manifold Effects of Positive Affect on Heart Rate Variability in Everyday Life: Distinguishing Within-Person and Between-Person Associations." *Health Psychology* 33(9): 1065.

Sherlin, L., F. Muench, and S. Wyckoff. 2010. "Respiratory Sinus Arrhythmia Feedback in a Stressed Population Exposed to a Brief Stressor Demonstrated by Quantitative EEG and sLORETA." *Applied Psychophysiological Biofeedback* 35: 219–228. doi:10.1007/s10484-010-9132-z

Siegmund, A., L. Köster, A. M. Meves, J. Plag, M. Stoy, and A. Ströhle. 2011. "Stress Hormones During Flooding Therapy and Their Relationship to Therapy Outcome in Patients with Panic Disorder and Agoraphobia." *Journal of Psychiatric Research* 45(3): 339–346.

Stang, H., and D. Treleaven (host and guest) (2018, May 22) "Trauma-Sensitive Mindfulness with David Treleaven" (Audio Podcast). https://www.youtube .com/watch?v=CyvnTMIDl9U

Steffen, P. R., T. Austin, A. DeBarros, and T. Brown. 2017. "The Impact of Resonance Frequency Breathing on Measures of Heart Rate Variability, Blood Pressure, and Mood." *Frontiers in Public Health* 5: 222. doi:10.3389 /fpubh.2017.00222

Van der Kolk, B. A. 2014. *The Body Keeps the Score: Brain, Mind, and Body in the Healing of Trauma.* New York: Viking.

Wells, R., T. Outhred, J. A. Hethers, D. S. Quintana, and A. H. Kemp. 2012. "A Randomized-Controlled Trial of Single-Session Biofeedback Training on Performance Anxiety and Heart Rate Variability in Musicians." *PLOS ONE* 7(10). doi:10.1371/journal.pone.0046597

Wylie, M. S. 2004. "The Limits of Talk: Bessel van der Kolk Wants to Transform the Treatment of Trauma." *Psychotherapy Networker* 28: 30–41.

Young, K. D., R. Phillips, V. Zotev, W. C. Drevets, and J. Bodurka. 2014. "Self-Regulation of Amygdala Activity with Real-Time fMRI Neurofeedback in Patients with Depression." *Neuropsychopharmacology* 38: S198–S313.

Zotev, V., R. Phillips, K. D. Young, W. C. Drevets, and J. Bodurka. 2013. "Prefrontal Control of the Amygdala During Real-Time fMRI Neurofeedback Training of Emotion Regulation." *PLOS ONE* 8(11): e79184. doi:10.1371/journal.pone.0079184

Zucker, T. L., K. W. Samuelson, F. Muench, M. A. Greenberg, and R. N. Gevirtz. 2009. "The Effects of Respiratory Sinus Arrhythmia Biofeedback on Heart Rate Variability and Posttraumatic Stress Disorder Symptoms: A Pilot Study." *Applied Psychophysiological Biofeedback* 34: 135–143. doi:10.1007/s10484-009-9085-2

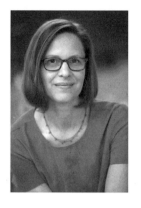

Rebekkah LaDyne, MS, SEP, is a somatic therapist, researcher, mind-body skills educator, and author. She is a member of the United States Association for Body Psychotherapy. Based on her extensive research in mind-body medicine at Saybrook University, her comprehensive training with the Somatic Experiencing® Trauma Institute, and her more than two decades of work in the field of embodied well-being, she developed the mind-body reset (MBR) protocol. Rebekkah has supported thousands of people, beginning from within her own wellness center, to groups she taught at Spirit Rock Meditation Center, and while traveling to worldwide destinations offering workshops and retreats. She has recorded several wellness CDs, appears on the radio and YouTube, and meets with clients online from all over the globe. She is in private practice in the San Francisco Bay Area where she lives with her husband and two daughters. She can be found online at www.rebekkahladyne.com.

Foreword writer **Kathy L. Kain, PhD,** has been practicing and teaching bodywork and trauma recovery for more than three decades. A senior trainer in Somatic Experiencing®, she is an expert in integrating touch into the practice of psychotherapy and trauma recovery, as well as in somatic approaches to working with developmental and complex trauma. She is coauthor of *Nurturing Resilience*.

Real change *is* possible

For more than forty-five years, New Harbinger has published proven-effective self-help books and pioneering workbooks to help readers of all ages and backgrounds improve mental health and well-being, and achieve lasting personal growth. In addition, our spirituality books offer profound guidance for deepening awareness and cultivating healing, self-discovery, and fulfillment.

Founded by psychologist Matthew McKay and Patrick Fanning, New Harbinger is proud to be an independent, employee-owned company. Our books reflect our core values of integrity, innovation, commitment, sustainability, compassion, and trust. Written by leaders in the field and recommended by therapists worldwide, New Harbinger books are practical, accessible, and provide real tools for real change.

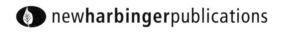 **newharbinger**publications

MORE BOOKS *from*
NEW HARBINGER PUBLICATIONS

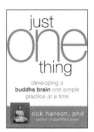
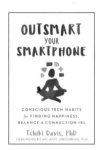
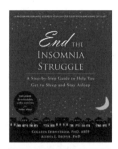
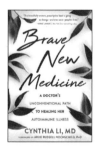
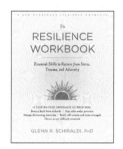
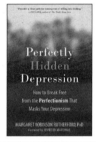
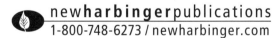